"One of the most creatively, physically fit people I kno[w] Suzy Chaffee makes a unique contribution to every s[ituation she] enters. Her book can help you take care of yourself in a way that's fun as well as good for you."

—DONNA DE VARONA
Olympic gold medalist

"Suzy has been the champion of rights and opportunities for athletes in the United States and the world, while maintaining her own championship form. Her book shares her secrets and includes some valuable flexibility exercises for men."

—BRUCE JENNER

"Suzy Chaffee has served on four Presidents' councils on physical fitness and has been a pioneer of the sports revolution in America. Suzy brings intelligence, fun, beauty, and soul to the image of fitness."

—GEORGE ALLEN
Chairman of the President's
Council on Physical Fitness

"When I went skiing with Suzy in Vail her skiing was surpassed only by her knowledge of the benefits of fitness and nutrition."

—PRESIDENT GERALD FORD

"Suzy Chaffee is a great athlete who has pioneered making exercise fun, effective, and interesting. It's so important that women develop more strength and men more flexibility to have a well-rounded fitness program. Right on, Suzy!"

—BILLIE JEAN KING

"I love New York and I love feeling physically fit. If this book will help me to ski like Suzy, I'll start tomorrow."

—CATHY LEE CROSBY

THE I ♥ NEW YORK FITNESS BOOK

April 28/83

To Sunny,
I owe you these pictures, coach,
and so much in life
My favorite douche bag
in love and crime.

♡

SUZY

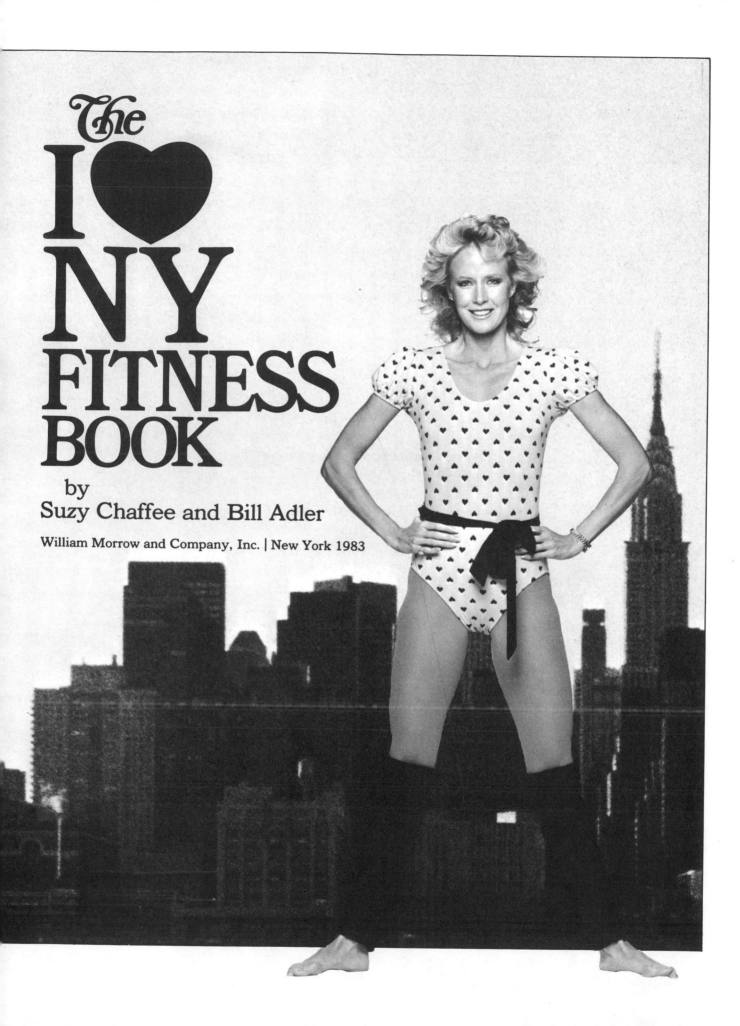

The
I ♥ NY
FITNESS
BOOK

by
Suzy Chaffee and Bill Adler

William Morrow and Company, Inc. | New York 1983

Grateful acknowledgment is extended to the following
for permission to use their photographs:

Marvin Newman,
for the silhouette photograph on page 14.

Robert Troxell,
for the ski photograph on page 18.

Peter Beard,
for the jogging photograph on page 220.

Library of Congress Catalog Card Number: 83-60414

ISBN: 0-688-02040-2

Printed in the United States of America

First Edition

1 2 3 4 5 6 7 8 9 10

Exterior photography: Vera Anderson

Interior photography: Joel Brodsky

Suzy's outfits designed by Stevi Brooks

To my mom for giving me the example of fitness, to my father for teaching me practical nutrition through his fruit and vegetable garden, to my brothers for their competition, to Sunny for her friendship, to all those who have given me love and support—and to everybody who cares about fitness

• ACKNOWLEDGMENTS •

We, and all America, owe a great debt to these fitness pioneers who have helped, and continue to help, keep our country healthy and strong: Bob Anderson, Walter Camp, Dr. Kenneth Cooper, Jacques D'Amboise, Donna de Verona, John Devlin, Jim Fixx, Ron Fletcher, Jane Fonda, Tim Gallaway, Billie Jean King, Nick Kounovsky, Jack La Lanne, George Leonard, Dan Lurie, Judy Massit, Joseph Pilate, Bonnie and Suzy Prudden, Arnold Schwarzenegger, Dr. George Sheehan, Ray Siegner, Richard Simmons, Jackie Sorenson, Kathy Switzer, Bob Uram, the teachers of the complete spectrum of fitness/nutrition throughout the land, the President's Council on Physical Fitness and Sports, the Women's Sports Foundation, and the numerous corporations who have sponsored fitness programs for their employees and the general public.

· SPECIAL THANKS TO ·

Elizabeth Frost Knappman, our editor; Cheryl Asherman, our art director; Liney Li, our book designer; and Betsy Cenedella, our copy editor, for their painstaking care and brilliance.

A fit person
is an advanced artist
bringing the joy of the feelings
into
the activity of the body.

—Suzy Chaffee

A note of caution:

Before beginning this, or any other, exercise program, it is advisable to obtain the approval and recommendations of your physician. While you're on this, or any, exercise program, it is advisable to visit your physician for periodic monitoring. This program is intended for adults in good health.

Contents

Why

This Book Is for

You

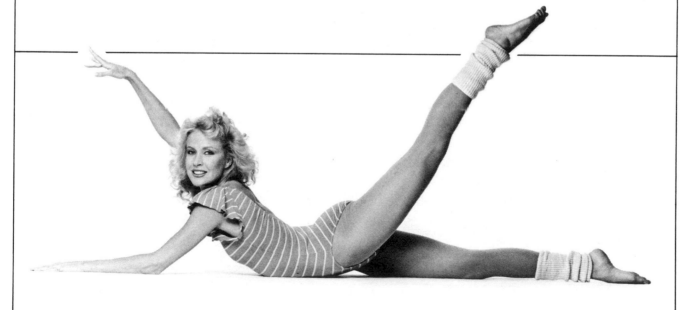

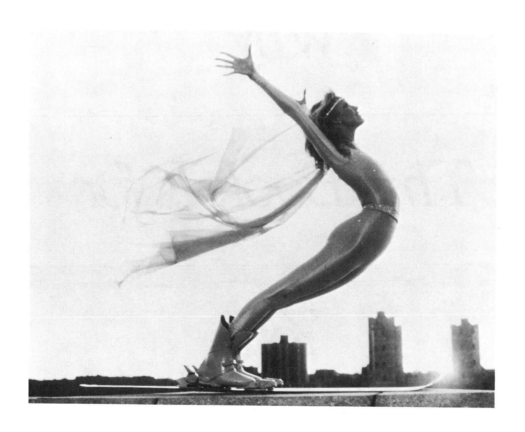

I love New York, and that's why I created this total fitness program: to live to my fullest under New York's stresses, tensions, excitements, and challenges. If you can keep it together in the Big Apple, you can feel just as healthy, brimming with life, and on top of the world in Anyplace, U.S.A. So this book is for you wherever you are—to make you feel terrific, and look as terrific as you feel.

I'm Suzy Chaffee, and all my life seems to have been a preparation for this book.

I put on my first pair of skis when I was two-and-a-half years old, and I've had a love affair with sports and fitness ever since. I have been the Number 1 ski racer, male or female, in the United States; captain of our Women's Olympic Ski Team; pioneer and three-time world champion in free-style skiing, a new sport that I helped invent. I play tennis and golf, run, swim, dance (disco, classical ballet, jazz, and my favorite: snow dancing on skis), roller- and ice-skate, ride horses, wind-surf, and, of course, work out daily.

I'm a fitness activist, and for a good part of the last fourteen years I've been telling the American people about exercise and nutrition. Working with many of the major health promotion groups—the President's Council on Physical Fitness and Sports is just one—I've carried a special message all over the nation. It's this: The human body—yours and mine—is a great work of art, the greatest ever conceived, and should be treated as such, with respect, with care, with love.

In this book, to make that message practical, I draw on all my experience of being fit and teaching fitness. Here is a total fitness program that is as pleasurable as it is do-able, that will work for you now and for the rest of your life. And it's a program that's like no fitness program you've ever been in or heard of before, because:

It's my way of feeling high while you burn away fat and sculpture your body into sensual sleekness.

It's my way of expressing yourself aesthetically while you prepare your body to perform at its peak in all of life's activities—from shopping to sports, from making money to making love.

It's my way of turning "dead time" into "live time" throughout your day, even when you're lying in bed or waiting for the toast to pop.

Above all, it's my way to good looks, good health, and good times.

Your goal is the same as mine: to see in your mirror a person you can view with love and pride. I've achieved this goal. So can you—with *The I Love New York Fitness Book.*

I'm a small-town girl, born in Rutland, Vermont, and brought up close to nature, which I love. That's my mother, an alternate on our Olympic Ski Team, who inspired me. The boys are my older brothers, Rick and Kim. Kim (left) went on to become captain of the Harvard Ski Team; and Rick, captain of two Olympic ski teams. Keeping up with them wasn't easy. But I did it, and still stayed feminine.

The two other members of my family don't appear in this picture—my father because he took it, and my younger brother, Mark, because he wasn't born yet. My father was a ski pioneer, and redheaded Mark grew up into a jock of all sports. Skiing and fitness kept our family together in more ways than one. It was not only fun, but it helped my brothers and me to become healthy, happy, and successful human beings.

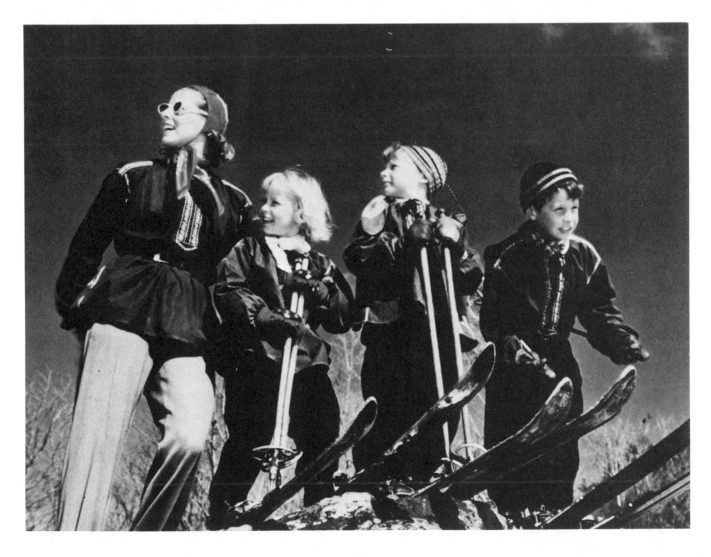

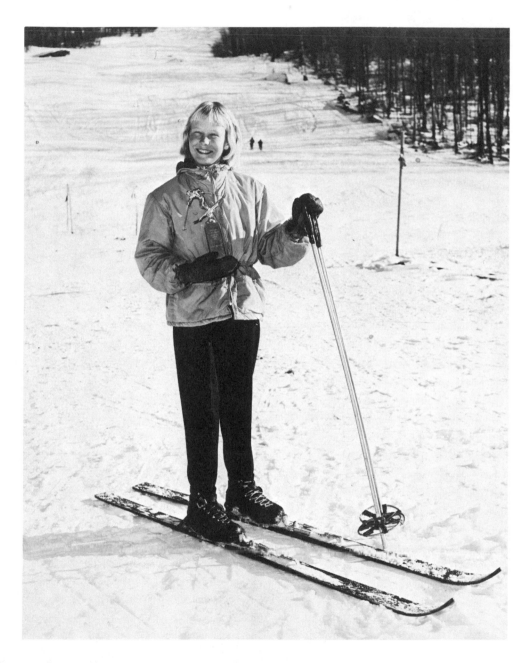

Aged ten, and winner of my first trophy (Eastern Junior Champion). There's nothing more thrilling than a peak performance. You feel invincible; nothing can go wrong. It's a natural high you'll never forget. But you don't have to win a championship to experience it. You can enjoy it every day of your life as you master the exercises in this book. My daily little victories are just as important as the big ones. Yours can be too.

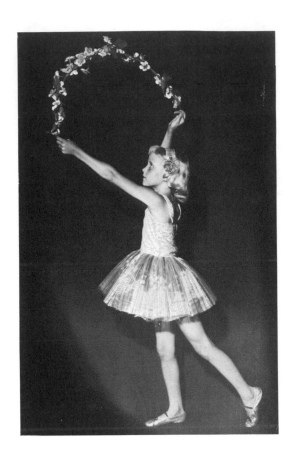

One of the features that sets my fitness program apart is its emphasis on graceful movements of the body. Here I am in my first tutu learning the basics of beautiful body motions, then later on expressing on skis the joy of gracefulness. The gracefulness you acquire from my exercises will make you more attractive in everything you do—and you don't have to start learning at the age of six.

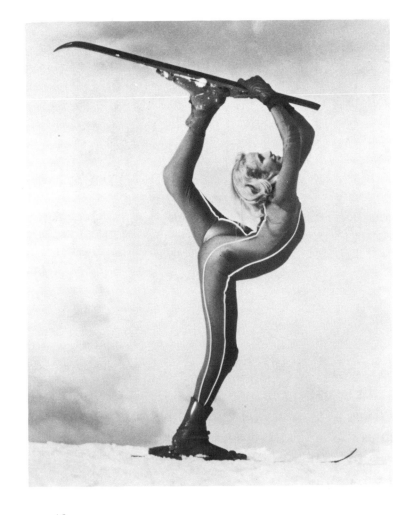

What The

I Love New York Fitness

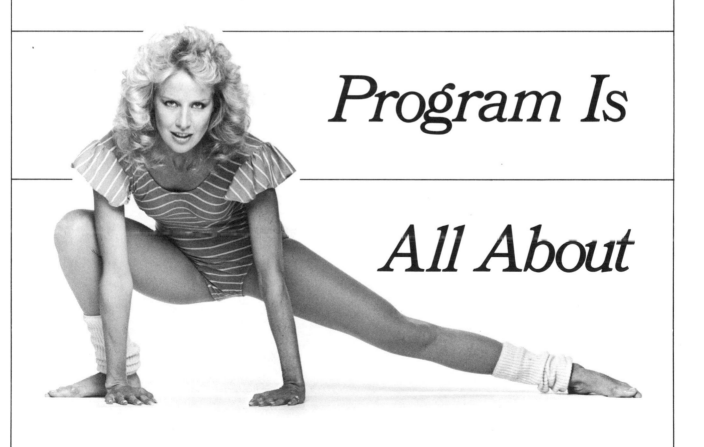

Program Is

All About

As a television personality and as an actress and model, I learned a universal truth when I appeared in front of a camera: Keep it simple.

I've kept this program so simple that you can enjoy it, benefit from it, and—most important—stick with it, even though you've never exercised regularly before.

You start with *Pretty Exercises* that put you on the fast track to bringing out the best in you, then push on to *Beautiful* and *Gorgeous Exercises* which are more demanding but more rewarding.

If on some days you can't find the time to do these exercises, switch to my *Anywhere, Anytime Exercises*. They're quickies you can fit in on your busiest day.

You can supplement my basic program with *Exercises with the Man in Your Life*. Try them, and thrill to a new kind of intimacy in your love life.

And if you're over fifty, don't despair—you can help turn the clock back to youthful slimness and good looks with my *Exercises for Super-Moms*. Flip to the proof on page 211. The model looks decades younger than her actual seventy. I know that's her true age because she's *my* Super-Mom.

All my exercises are feminine, fun, and fashionable. When you do a Suzy Chaffee original, it's like being in *Vogue* or *Cosmo* or *Bazaar*.

That's it.

The whole program.

As I said:

Simple.

Getting

Ready

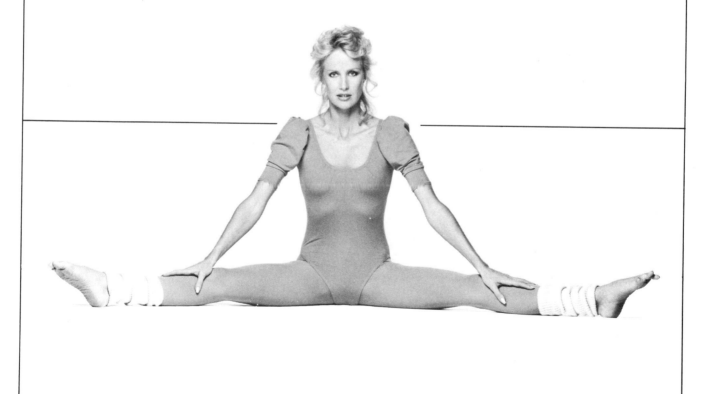

Beautiful Posture—and How to Develop It

If you are not already blessed with perfect posture, awareness of your posture weaknesses is the first step toward that blessing. Poor posture affects your whole body, puts stress on your skeleton and internal organs, works against your sports performance, and damages your self-image. I used to have terrible posture, and here's how I figured out how to correct it. And—wow!—did it work! So why not start by making a posture check right now? Best way is to take off your clothes, stand in front of a full-length mirror, and see if you have any of these faults.

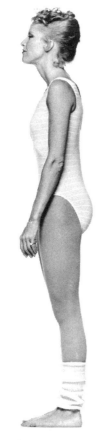 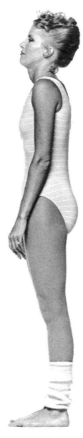 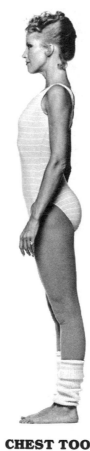 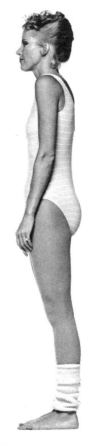

HEAD TOO FAR FORWARD   **HEAD TOO FAR BACK**   **CHEST TOO FAR FORWARD**   **CHEST DROPPED**

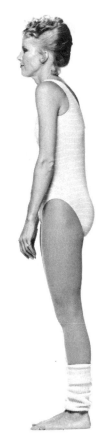 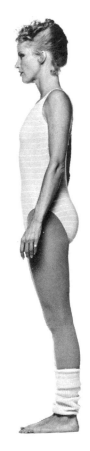 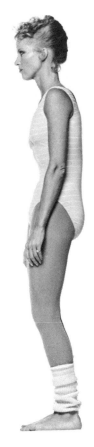 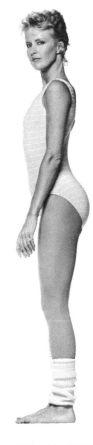

SHOULDERS TOO FAR FORWARD   **SHOULDERS TOO FAR BACK**   **BACK ROUNDED**   **BACK ARCHED**

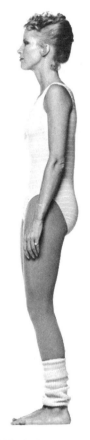 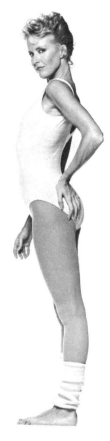 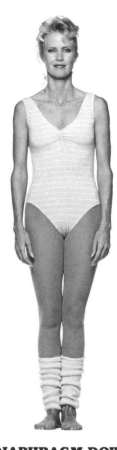 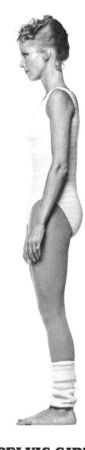

| PELVIS TILTED FORWARD | PELVIS TILTED BACKWARD | DIAPHRAGM DOWN | PELVIC GIRDLE (STOMACH AND BUTTOCKS) TOO LOOSE |

Compare your weaknesses with the following illustration of perfect posture. It shows the proper way to hold your diaphragm up; pelvic girdle tight; and pelvis, head, chest, and shoulders centered.

Then try my exaggeration-awareness exercises. The idea is to exaggerate your weaknesses, then correct them, and see the stunning difference. For example, if your head is too far forward, hold it *way* forward, then *way* back; then center it. How wonderful you look on center! Then close your eyes and *feel* the difference. Try the exaggeration-awareness exercise for each of your weaknesses.

Awareness is the first step. Then, by practicing the exercises in the following chapters regularly, you'll strengthen your posture muscles to create naturally beautiful body lines.

With proper posture, you won't walk this way (as I used to do):

You'll walk elegantly.

Practice walking in front of a full-length mirror until you feel smooth and relaxed. Then walking elegantly, with an air of casual confidence, will become a natural part of your life.

Warmups

These preliminary exercises are going to warm up your body by speeding up the action of your heart and lungs, and gently limbering up your muscles. That will reduce the possibility of unnecessary strain, and prepare you for the greater exertion needed for conditioning exercises.

For starters, repeat each exercise only five times, and between exercises relax and take a breather if you feel the need. (Rushing things may make your body rebel with aches and pains.) Then, from day to day, gradually increase the number of repetitions (you'll know you've reached maximum when you feel a slight burn). Gradually increasing the number of repetitions will continue to improve your agility, flexibility, and endurance.

I warm up with aerobic and stretch exercises, spending at least three minutes on each of them.

• AEROBIC WARMUPS •

The object here is to get your blood flowing better through your heart and muscles. Blood carries oxygen which nourishes and invigorates the tissues. With aerobic exercises, you tense and relax your muscles rhythmically, and that speeds the blood flow.

The American Heart Association recommends aerobic exercises because they promote the health of your heart and the blood vessels associated with it (the cardiovascular system). These warmups could help you live longer, without the fear of heart attack. So when you do these exercises, put your heart into them.

Correct Breathing

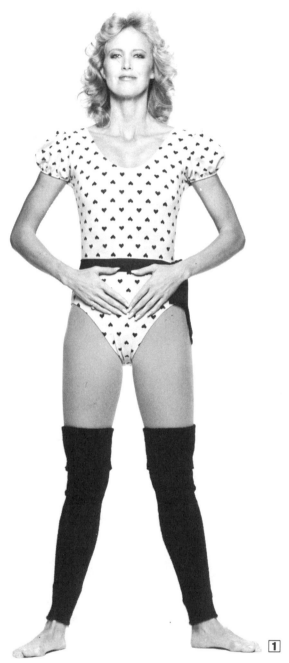

1 Stand erect. Bend your elbows, place your palms against your stomach, and relax your shoulders, throat, face, and chest.

2 Inhale through your nose, and feel your stomach going out.

3 Exhale through your mouth with a whooshing sound, and feel your stomach going in.

Breathing correctly not only brings in the maximum amount of air but also strengthens your stomach muscles. These breathing ex-ercises alone can, in the long run, give you that attractive flat stomach you've always wanted.

Breathe correctly through every aerobic exercise. It's excellent practice for breathing correctly through *all* your exercises.

Jog in Place

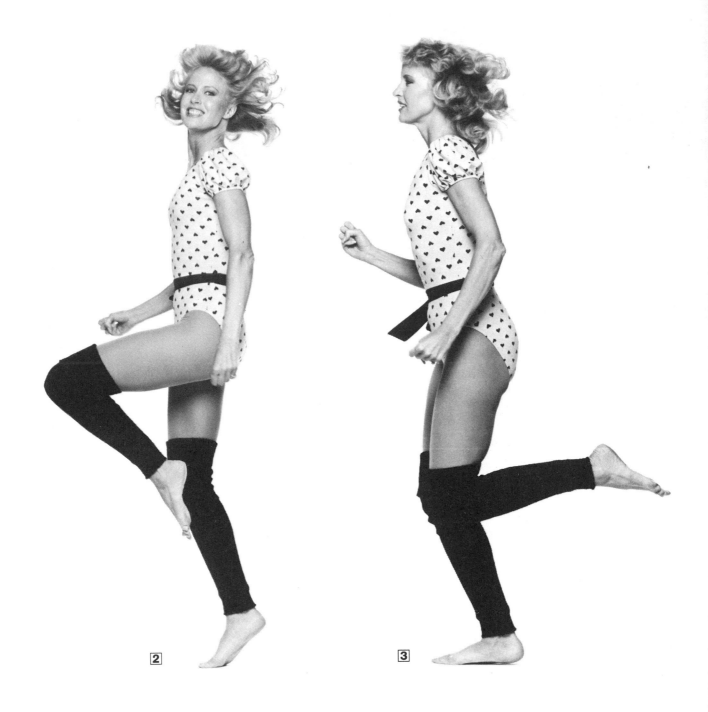

1 Jog in place, swinging your arms freely and landing on the balls of your feet, then your heels.

2 Jog with knees up high.

3 Jog, kicking your heels up high.

Jumping for Joy

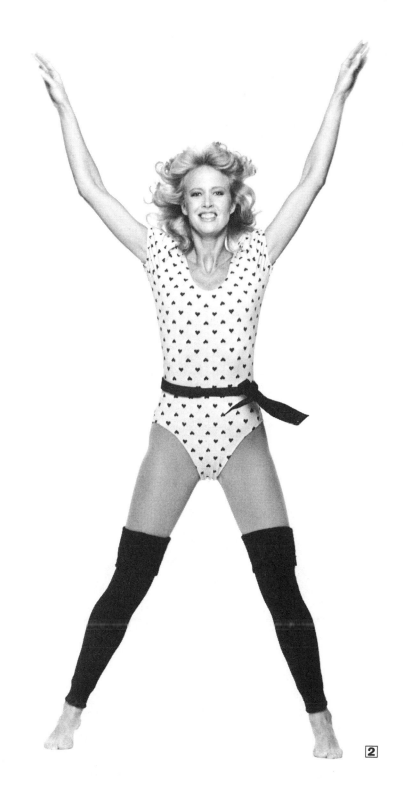

2

1 Stand erect, feet to-gether, arms at sides.

2 Jump, spreading your legs apart and flinging your arms upward at an angle away from your head.

3 Jump back to starting position, and repeat.

33

Twist

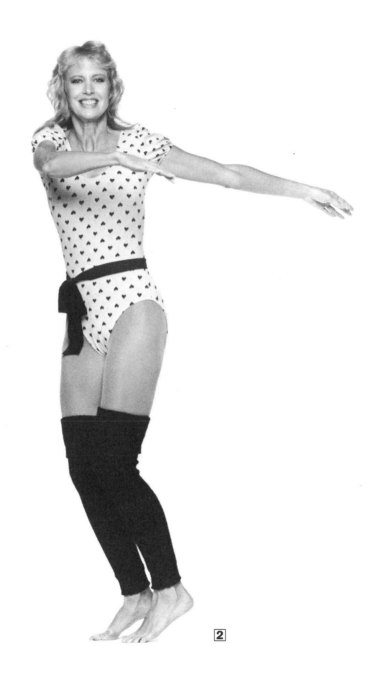

2

1 Stand erect, arms at sides, legs together.

2 On the balls of your feet, twist as if doing the dance. As your right hip swivels forward, swing your arms to the left, right arm bent across your body and left arm out straight.

3 Reverse, bringing your left hip forward and swinging your arms across to the right.

The Slalom

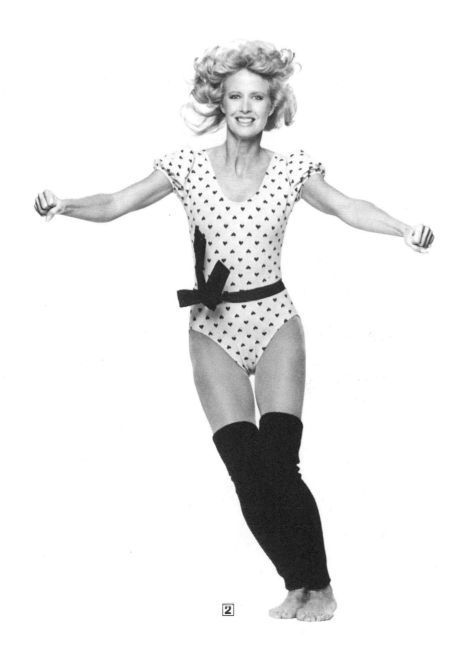

1 Stand erect, with your legs together and your arms out straight to the sides, inclined slightly downward and forward for balancing, as if you were holding ski poles.

2 Bend your knees and ankles, and jump from side to side as if you were leaping over obstacles.

Note: For extra balance in this exercise, and all balancing exercises, tense your arms just as you would if you were hugging a big teddy bear. Applying this arm tension technique can help your balance in many sports.

One-Leg Kicks

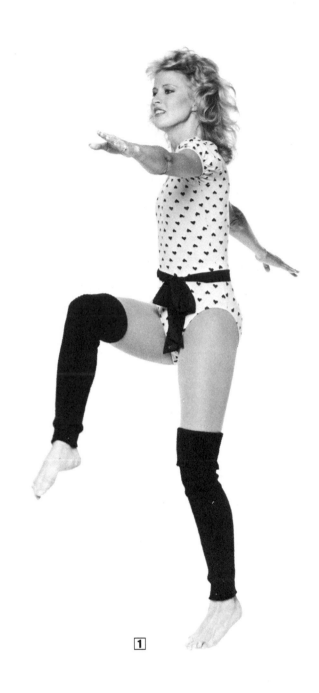

1 Stand on your left leg with the knee slightly bent, arms extended to the sides. Your right leg should be lifted diagonally to the left, knee bent to the left, toes pointed.

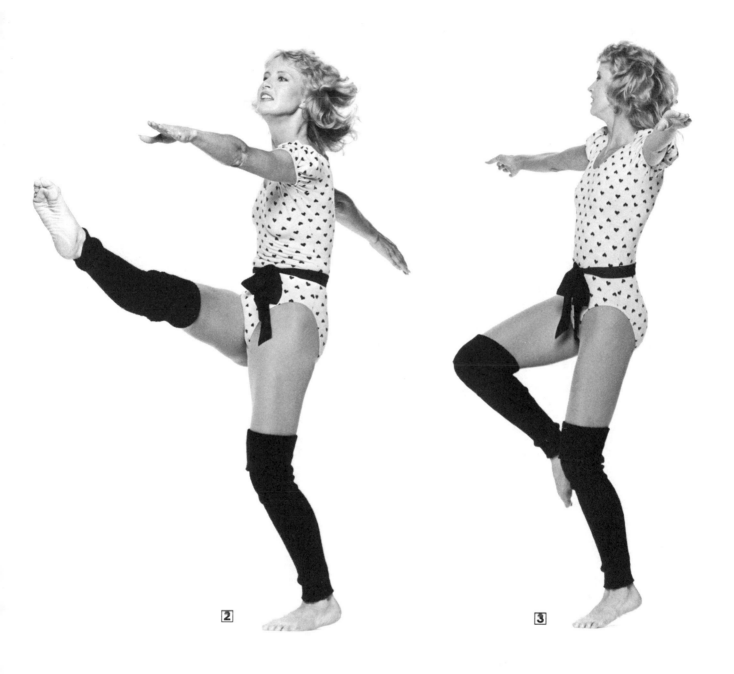

2   Kick your right leg as high as you can.

3   Bend your right leg, touching your left knee with the sole of your right foot.

4   Repeat, this time kicking to the right. Keep alternating the direction of your kicks.

Now try it standing on your right leg and kicking with your left.

Kick Claps

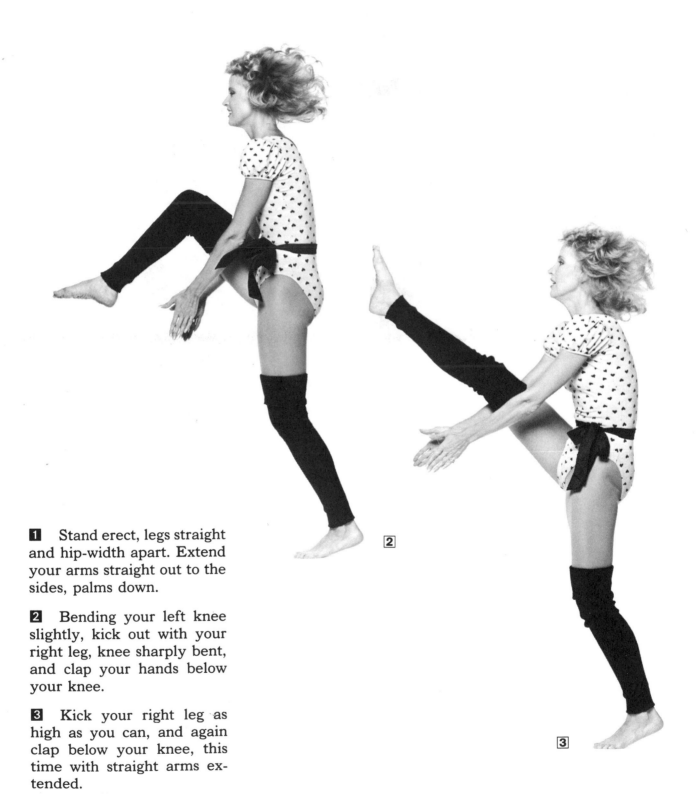

1 Stand erect, legs straight and hip-width apart. Extend your arms straight out to the sides, palms down.

2 Bending your left knee slightly, kick out with your right leg, knee sharply bent, and clap your hands below your knee.

3 Kick your right leg as high as you can, and again clap below your knee, this time with straight arms extended.

4 Repeat, kicking with left leg; then continue, alternating legs.

Vaudeville

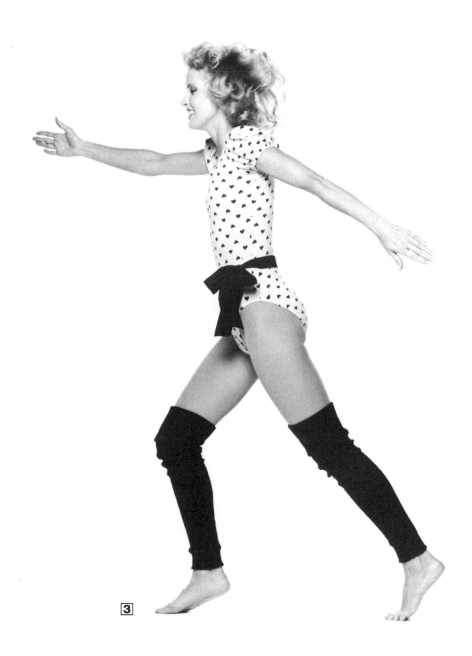

1 Stand erect, feet together, hands at sides.

2 Take a long stride forward on your left leg, bending the knee, while standing on the toes of your right leg, left arm extended straight ahead, right arm extended back diagonally.

3 Now stride forward with your right leg, bending the knee, while standing on the toes of your left leg, right arm extended straight ahead, left arm extended back diagonally.

4 Continue these strides with increased tempo, and you'll feel like an old-time vaudevillian strutting across the stage.

Cross Legs

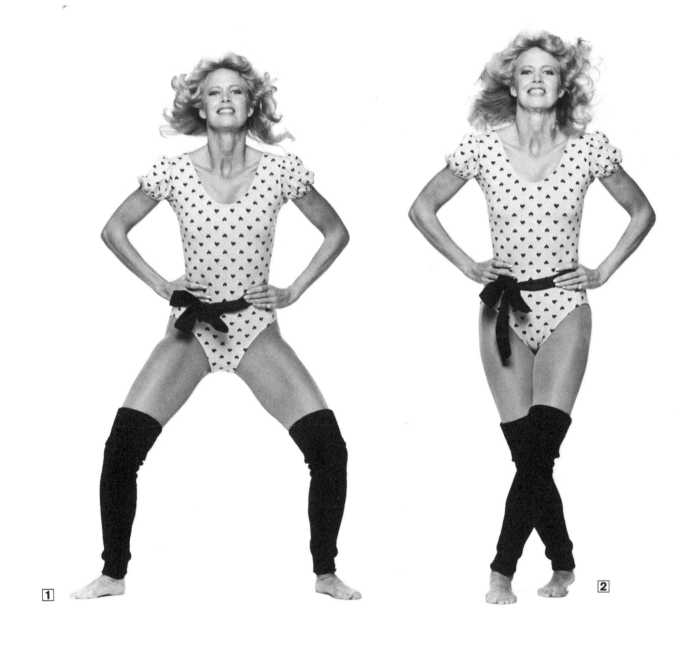

1 Stand with legs wide apart, knees bent outward, arms akimbo, hands touching waist.

2 Cross your left leg over the right. Return to starting position; then cross the right over the left, and continue at increasing speed.

Side Swings

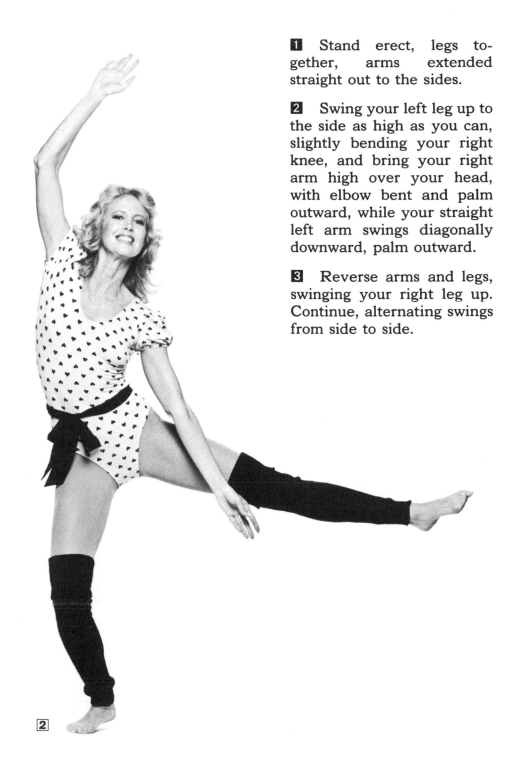

1 Stand erect, legs together, arms extended straight out to the sides.

2 Swing your left leg up to the side as high as you can, slightly bending your right knee, and bring your right arm high over your head, with elbow bent and palm outward, while your straight left arm swings diagonally downward, palm outward.

3 Reverse arms and legs, swinging your right leg up. Continue, alternating swings from side to side.

• STRETCH WARMUPS •

Once your body is warmed up through aerobic exercises, you can s–t–r–e–t–c–h until you feel a gentle pull. You'll be delighted by how those tight muscles begin to loosen up, and feel free. That's what these stretch warmups are all about.

Head Rolls

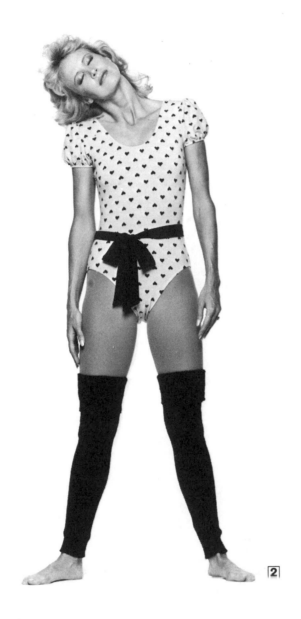

1 Stand with your feet about hip-width apart and pointing diagonally outward, arms at sides, fingers loose. Keep your shoulders down and relaxed.

2 Roll your head clockwise 180 degrees, stretching your neck as far as you can toward each shoulder.

3 Roll your head in the opposite direction 180 degrees and continue, alternating directions.

Shoulder Circles

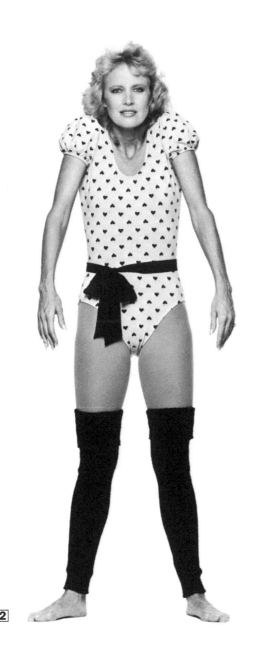

2

1 Stand with your feet about hip-width apart and pointing diagonally outward, arms slightly out from your sides, fingers loose.

2 Lift your shoulders as close to your ears as you can, and swivel them back and forward several times.

3 Bring your shoulders up and forward in a circular motion.

Repeat.

Shoulder Back Twist

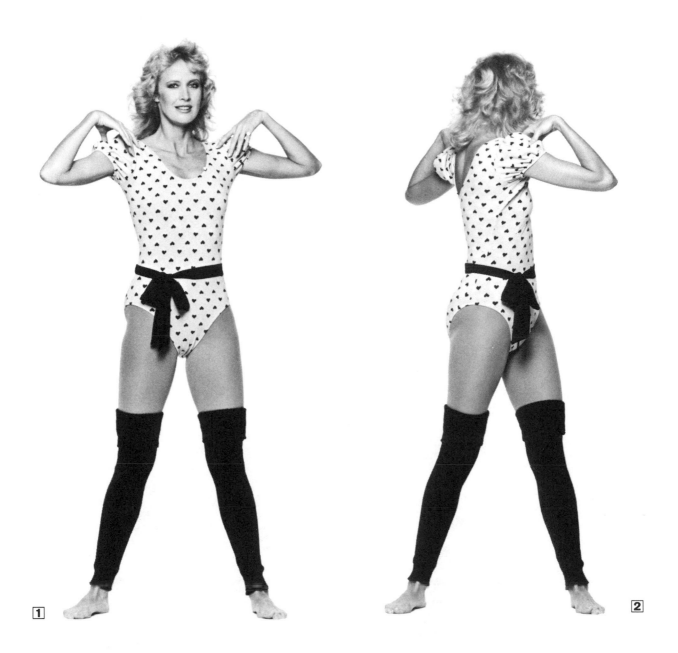

1 Stand with your feet about hip-width apart and pointing diagonally forward, arms to the sides with elbows bent and fingers spread loosely on your shoulders. Your fingers and wrist should form an inverted V.

2 Twist back, and look around as far behind you as possible, first in one direction, then in the other.

Repeat.

Back Stretch

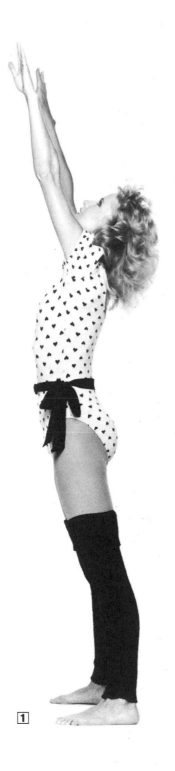

1 Stand with your feet about hip-width apart and pointing outward. Stretch your arms straight up, fingers spread.

2 Keeping your knees straight, roll your torso forward and down, and extend your arms back between your legs as far as they can go.

Repeat.

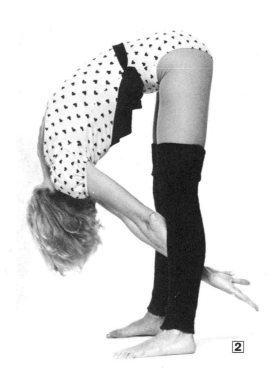

1

2

Ham Stretch

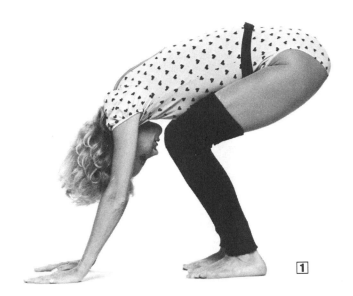

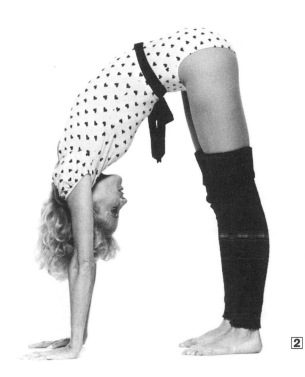

Ham is short for the hamstring muscles on the inner side of the thigh.

1 Standing with legs close together and knees bent, roll your torso forward until your chin is at knee level. Support yourself on straight arms inclined slightly forward, your palms flat on the floor, fingers pointing forward.

2 Straighten your legs and arch your back.

Repeat.

Hip Swivel

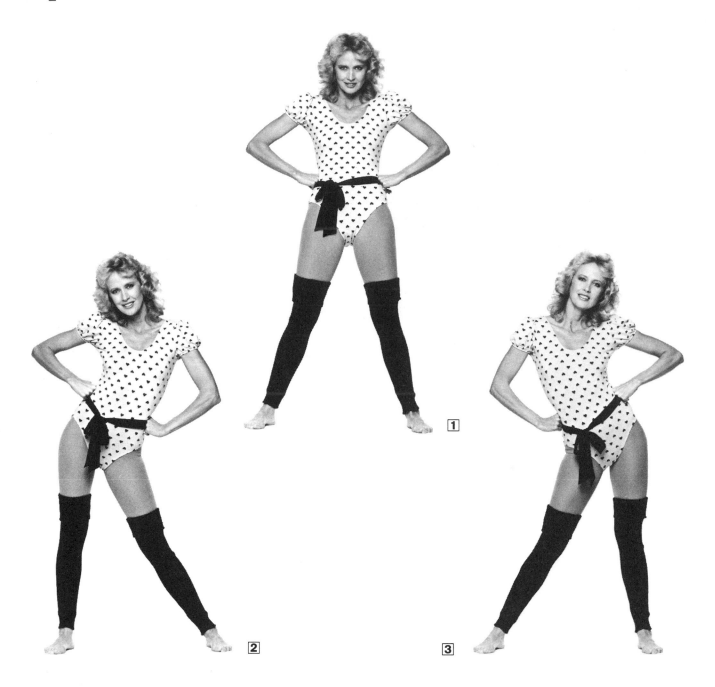

1 Standing, arms akimbo, extend your right hip to the right side. Your right leg should be straight and perpendicular to floor, your left leg extending diagonally.

2 Roll hips to center, extending your pelvis forward with the buttocks tight, legs straight and spread apart.

3 Roll hips to the left, with your left leg straight, your right leg extended diagonally.

4 Reverse steps 1 to 3 without stopping at the center position.

Repeat.

Knee Circles

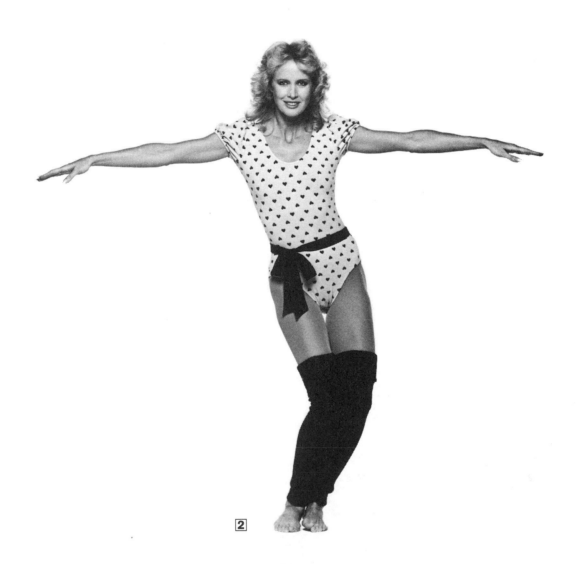

1 Stand with your legs together, feet pointing forward, and your arms extended straight out to the sides, palms down, fingers loose.

2 Bend your knees, keeping them together, and continuously pivot them clockwise and then counterclockwise.

Elbow to Ankle

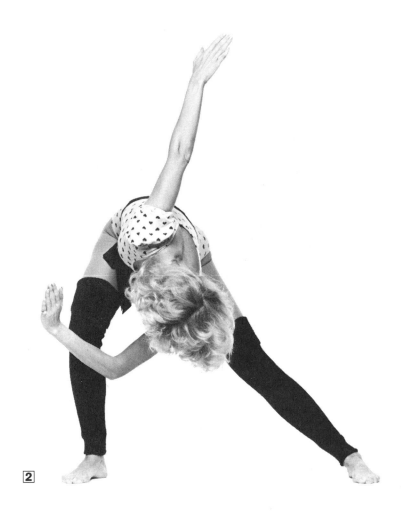

1 Stand erect, with your feet somewhat more than hip-width apart, your arms extended straight out to the sides, palms down, fingers together.

2 Bend forward, bending your left elbow, and bring it as close to your right ankle as you can.

3 Repeat with the right elbow, and continue to alternate sides.

Calf Stretch

1 With palms and feet flat on floor, both pointing forward, raise your buttocks up until your body forms an inverted V.

2 Keeping your left leg straight, heel flat on the floor, bring your right leg forward, knee bent, and distribute your weight between the ball of your right foot and the heel of your left. The stretch comes from putting the heel flat on the floor.

3 Repeat, bending your left knee, and continue to alternate sides.

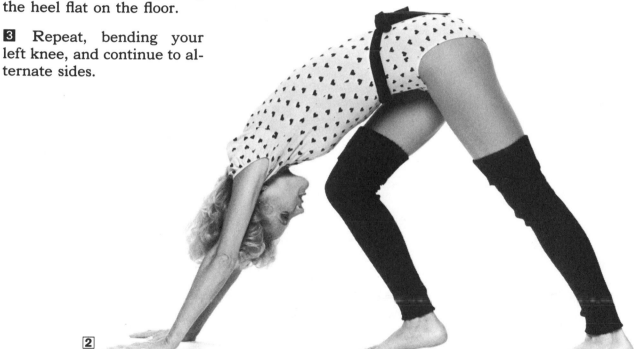

2

Hanging Roll Up

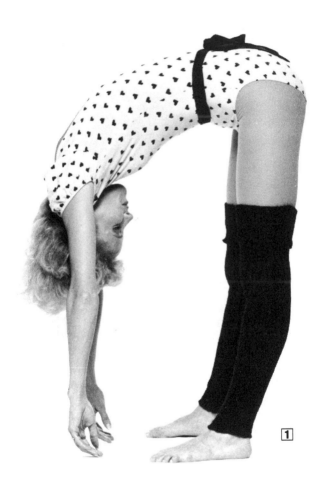

1 Bend from the waist as far as you can go, feet shoulder-width apart, arms dangling loosely.

2 Roll your torso up very slowly to erect position, with your arms straight up over your head, palms out.

The Flexibility Test

Flexibility is one of the most critical, yet underrated, goals of a well-rounded fitness program. That's why I invented this test, which is presented here for the first time. Take it after your warmups; then take it again after your first conditioning session, and you'll be astonished by the rise in your flexibility rating. It's instant encouragement, and that's what we all need when we start anything new.

Flexibility is even more a man's problem than a woman's. (*Your* toughest job is building more muscular strength.) But don't minimize the role a flexible body plays in your life. Lack of flexibility is a cause of lower-back pain, neck pain, charley horses, pains associated with running, and pulled and ripped ligaments and tendons. On the other hand, flexibility helps prevent injury while making you more supple, graceful, and attractive. And don't forget the Chaffee Law: The more flexible your body, the more flexible your mind.

Don't skip this test, because it's also an exercise—a curtain raiser that will whet your appetite for the dramatic experience in fitness ahead of you. And take the test regularly. Your score (which is based on how close you come to the goal set for you in each part of the test) is numerical proof that you're getting more and more flexible every day.

Toe Touch

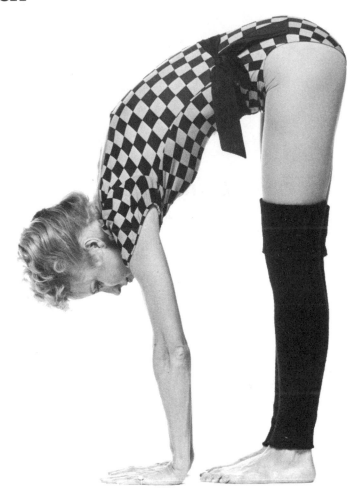

Stand erect, legs straight and together, feet pointing forward. Stretch up with your arms overhead; then bend down as far as you can. Your goal: to place your palms flat on the floor. Repeat; then test and score yourself.

Result	Points
Reach mid-calf	1
Reach ankle	2
Reach instep	3
Reach toes	4
Reach floor	5
Place hands flat on floor	6
YOUR SCORE:	

Back Twist

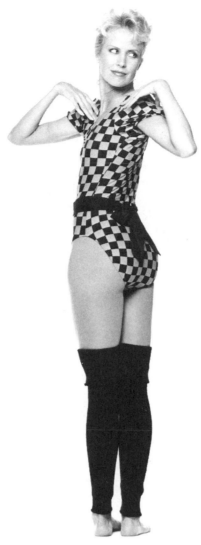

Stand erect, feet apart, hands on shoulders, elbows bent. Twist back around as far as you can go. Your goal: to see as far behind you as you can. Twist in both directions. Repeat; then test, averaging results.

Result	Points
See one-quarter way to directly behind you	1
See halfway to directly behind you	2
See three-quarters way to directly behind you	3
See directly behind you	4
See one-quarter more than directly behind you	5
See all the way around to the front (out of the corner of your eye)	6
YOUR SCORE:	

Leg Kicks

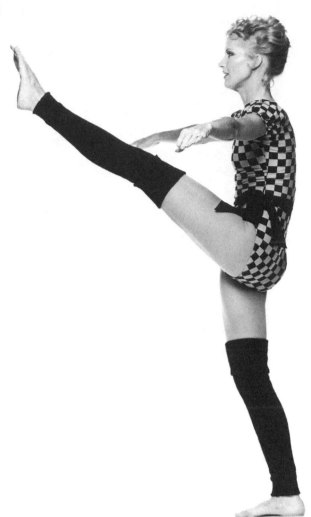

Stand on one leg, arms out to the sides for stability, and kick as high as you can. Your goal: to kick above your head. Repeat with the other leg; then test.

Result	Points
Kick hip-high	1
Kick waist-high	2
Kick chest-high	3
Kick shoulder-high	4
Kick head-high	5
Kick above head	6
YOUR SCORE:	

Side Stretch

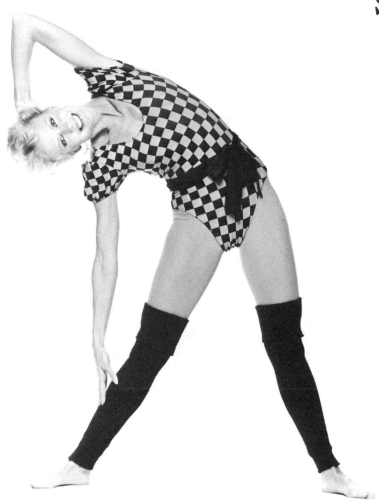

Stand erect, legs apart. Place one hand behind your neck, keeping your rib cage up and your knees locked straight, and reach down the side of your leg as far as you can go. Your goal: to touch just above the ankle. Repeat on the other side, and test.

Result	Points
Touch above knee	1
Touch knee	2
Touch upper calf	3
Touch mid-calf	4
Touch lower calf	5
Touch just above ankle	6
YOUR SCORE:	

Shoulder Stretch

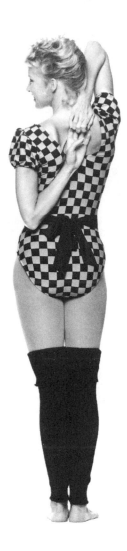

Use a mirror to observe your back. Stand erect, with one arm bent up behind your back as far as it will go, and the other arm bent from above, down your back. Try to bring your hands together. Your goal: to grasp fingers. Repeat from the other side; then test.

Result	Points
Fingers about 5 inches apart	1
Fingers about 3 inches apart	2
Fingers about 2 inches apart	3
Fingers about 1 inch apart	4
Fingers touching	5
Fingers grasped	6
YOUR SCORE:	

WHAT YOUR SCORE MEANS:

Add up your points for each exercise and divide by 5. If you averaged 6, you can be proud of your flexibility. If you averaged less than 6, you need more work; the lower your score, the more work you need. No matter how low your initial score, remember: Stick to this fitness program and you can make a perfect 6, which could easily lead to a perfect 10.

IV

The Pretty,

The Beautiful, and

The Gorgeous

Exercises

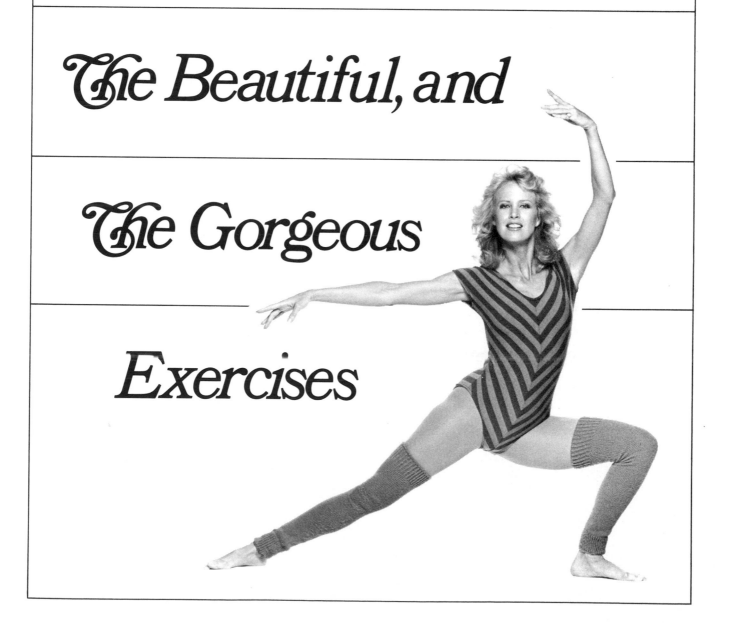

Why did I select those names for my exercises, instead of Beginners, Intermediate, and Advanced?

First, the negative reasons: I think the word *beginner* is a put-down. When I joined one of Jane Fonda's Beginners' classes (I recommend going to all kinds of classes for inspiration, as often as time permits), being labeled *beginner* made me feel so klutzy I acted klutzy. But in her *advanced* class, I felt like the most advanced.

We tend to live up to our labels; so why not live up to the labels *Pretty, Beautiful*, and *Georgeous*. Which is what I did—and that's how the Pretty, the Beautiful, and the Gorgeous Exercises were born.

Here's how to get the most out of these exercises:

Do them in the order in which they appear. They are planned to tone up systematically the muscles of your arms, abdomen, waist, buttocks, legs and hips, back, and the muscles controlling your balance.

Study the photographs and imitate the poses without deviation. (Later on, you can let yourself go and improvise to your heart's content, but not while you're learning.) Pay attention to details—the line of your hand, the straightness of your knees, the point of your toe, the tilt of your head. Almost from the start you'll find yourself performing aesthetically. Catch yourself in a full-length mirror and you'll want to applaud. Others watching you *will* applaud.

Pick a convenient time of day to start this program, and stick to it. I prefer mornings. If you leave it for later in the day, chances are you'll leave it out of your day. Exercising in the morning starts you off with an I-can-take-on-anything attitude—and that's how winners are made.

Repeat each exercise until you feel a "burn"—that's your body's signal to shake out your strongest muscle with relaxation between repeats, or even take a breather between exercises. As the days go by, gradually decrease the time of your breathing spells to zero. The object is to master the Pretty Exercises, then go on and do the same for the Beautiful and Gorgeous Exercises.

Your Flexibility Test ratings will point up your progress, but don't expect dramatic changes overnight. As the exercises give you attractive muscle tone, and increase flexibility and strength, the best in you will gradually be revealed. You'll move with smoothness and grace, and you'll look—well, that depends on how far you go with the program—even more pretty, or beautiful, or gorgeous than you are.

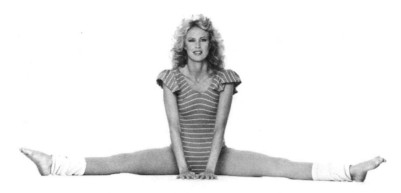

The Pretty Exercises

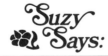

Arm Circles

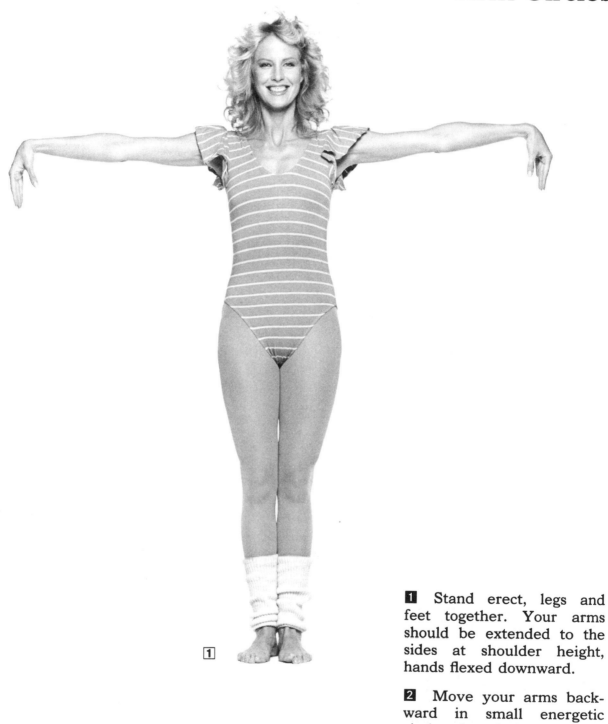

1 Stand erect, legs and feet together. Your arms should be extended to the sides at shoulder height, hands flexed downward.

2 Move your arms backward in small energetic circles, keeping your head erect.

3 Repeat, making forward circles.

Ballet Arms

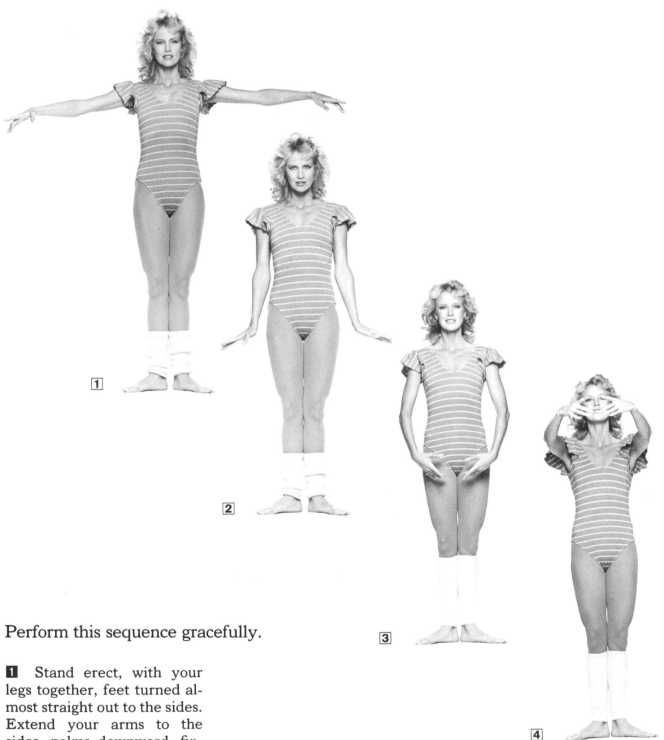

Perform this sequence gracefully.

1 Stand erect, with your legs together, feet turned almost straight out to the sides. Extend your arms to the sides, palms downward, fingers gracefully extended.

2 Bring your arms down parallel to and slightly out from your body, with your hands maintaining their former position.

3 Bending your elbows slightly, curve your arms and hands forward until your fingers are just a few inches apart in front of your body, about hip-high.

4 Maintaining the curve of your arms, raise them before you to chin height, fingers still almost touching.

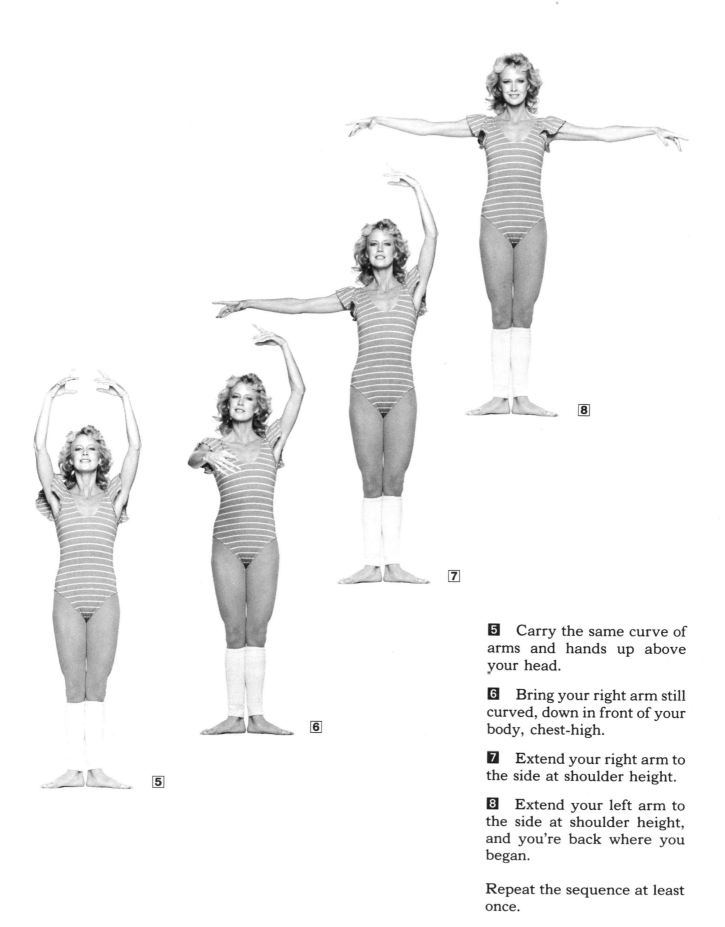

5 Carry the same curve of arms and hands up above your head.

6 Bring your right arm still curved, down in front of your body, chest-high.

7 Extend your right arm to the side at shoulder height.

8 Extend your left arm to the side at shoulder height, and you're back where you began.

Repeat the sequence at least once.

Shoulder Pulls (Upper)

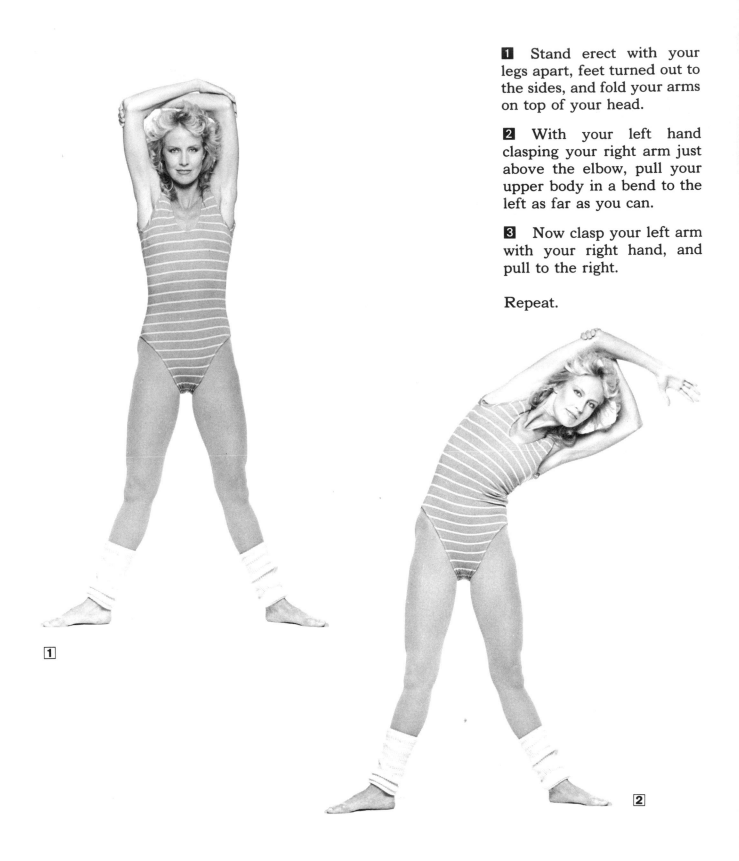

1 Stand erect with your legs apart, feet turned out to the sides, and fold your arms on top of your head.

2 With your left hand clasping your right arm just above the elbow, pull your upper body in a bend to the left as far as you can.

3 Now clasp your left arm with your right hand, and pull to the right.

Repeat.

Shoulder Pulls (Lower)

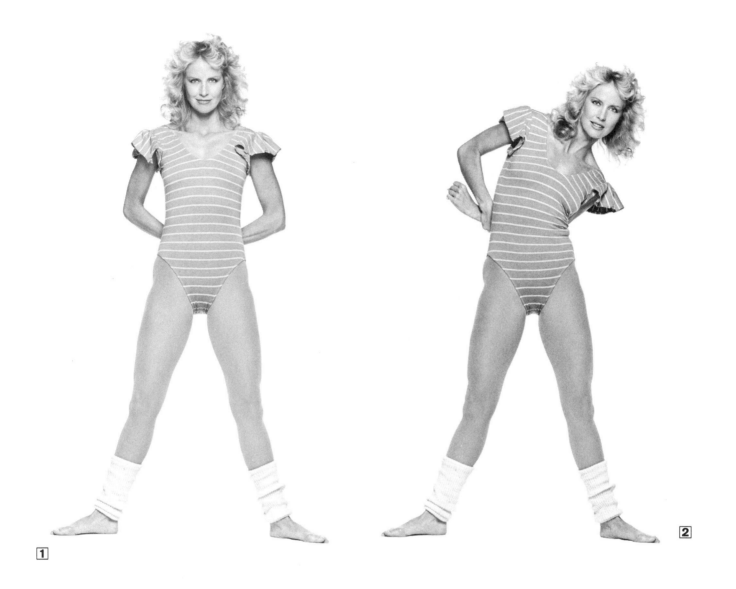

1   Stand erect, legs apart, feet turned out. Put your hands behind you at waist height, your right hand clasping your left wrist.

2   Pull your upper body in a bend to the left as far as you can.

3   Repeat, with your left hand clasping your right wrist and pulling your upper body to the left.

Back Arm Extension

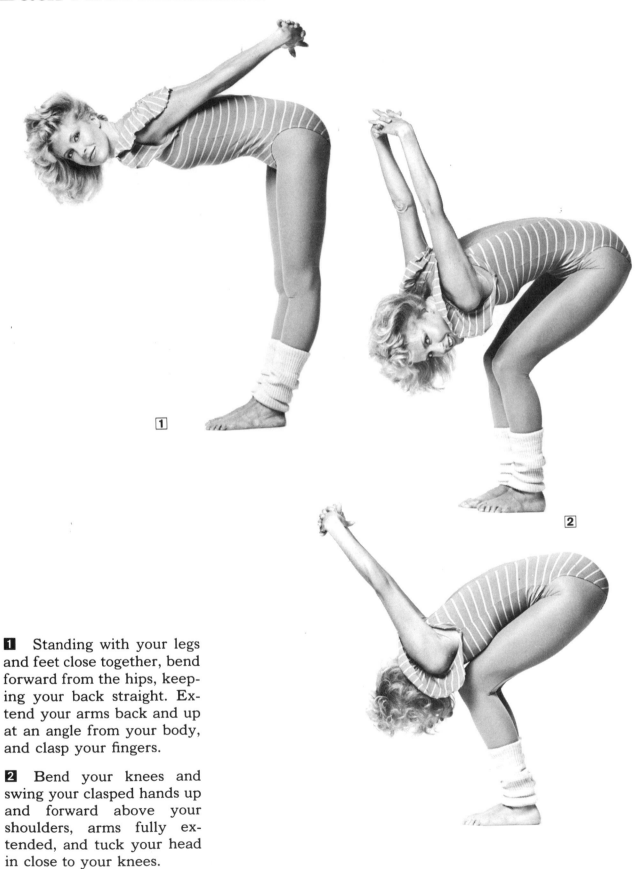

1 Standing with your legs and feet close together, bend forward from the hips, keeping your back straight. Extend your arms back and up at an angle from your body, and clasp your fingers.

2 Bend your knees and swing your clasped hands up and forward above your shoulders, arms fully extended, and tuck your head in close to your knees.

Froggy Ups

REGULAR

1 On spread knees, lean forward, keeping your body in a straight line from knees to head. Support yourself on your arms, with your hands pointing forward, a little more than shoulder-width apart. Raise your lower legs from the floor at a 45-degree angle, with the soles of your feet touching.

2 Bending your elbows and keeping your back straight, bring your body as close to the floor as you can.

3 Raise your body by straightening your arms, and repeat.

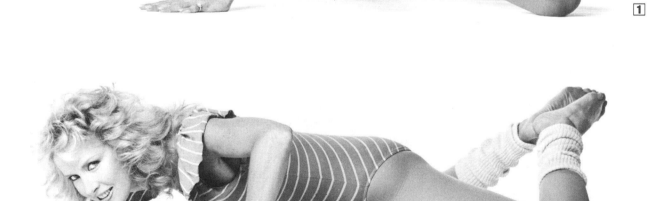

1

2

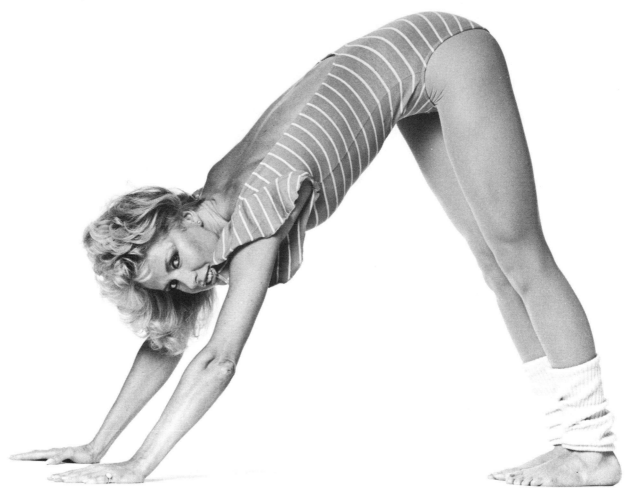

[1]

RELEASE

1 Standing with feet together and pointing forward, form an inverted V with your buttocks at the apex, supporting yourself on straight arms. Your hands should be shoulder-distance apart, pointing forward, with your palms flat on the floor, and your head between your arms.

2 Stretch your calf muscles by rocking back and forth.

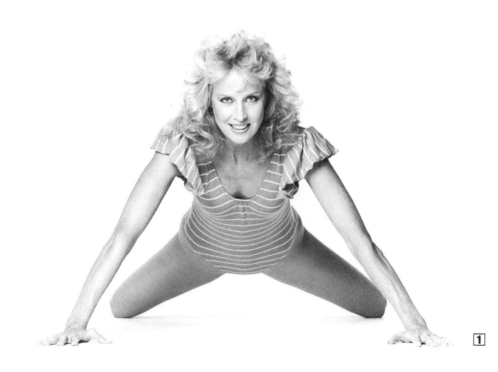

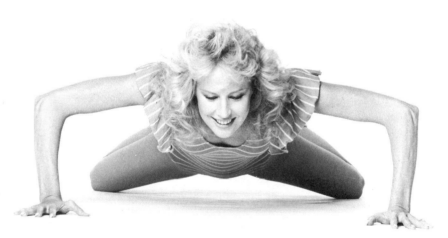

WIDE ARMS

1 Start in the same position as for Regular Froggy Ups, except that your arms should be spread wider.

2 Follow steps 2 and 3 of Regular Froggy Ups.

REPEAT RELEASE

73

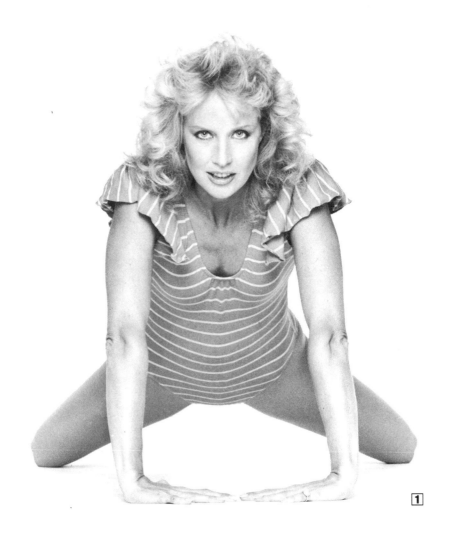

FINGERS TOGETHER

1 Vary the starting position of Regular Froggy Ups by placing your hands facing each other with the fingertips almost touching.

2 Follow steps 2 and 3 of Regular Froggy Ups.

REPEAT RELEASE

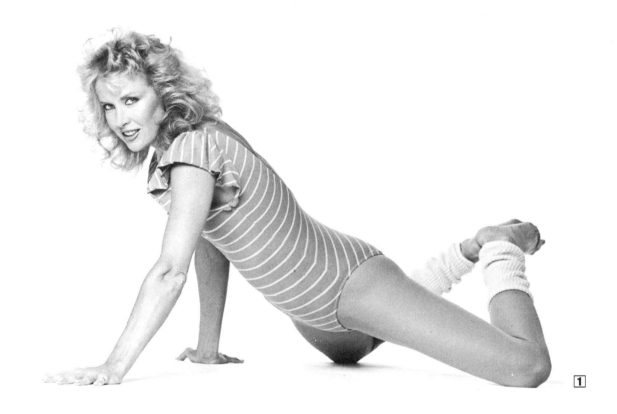

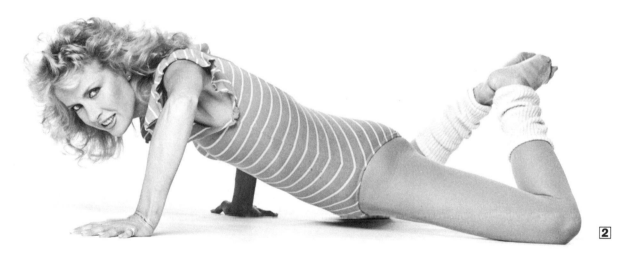

DIAGONALS

1 This time, the starting position of Regular Froggy Ups is altered by placing your left arm forward and your right arm back, to form a diagonal.

2 Repeat steps 2 and 3 of Regular Froggy Ups.

REPEAT RELEASE

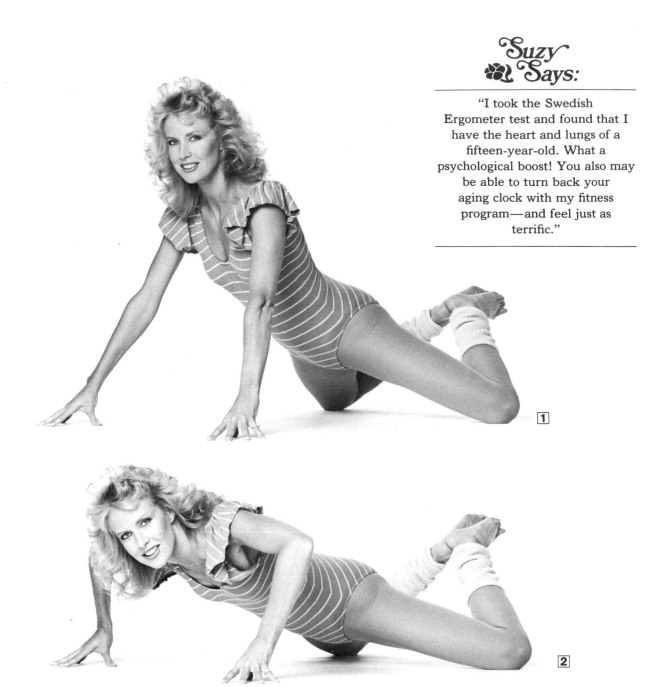

"I took the Swedish
Ergometer test and found that I
have the heart and lungs of a
fifteen-year-old. What a
psychological boost! You also may
be able to turn back your
aging clock with my fitness
program—and feel just as
terrific."

1

2

LADY FINGERS

1 Assume the same starting position as for Regular Froggy Ups, except support yourself on spread fingertips rather than on your palms.

2 Follow steps 2 and 3 of Regular Froggy Ups.

REPEAT RELEASE

Lower Abdominal

This exercise strengthens the lower abdominal muscles.

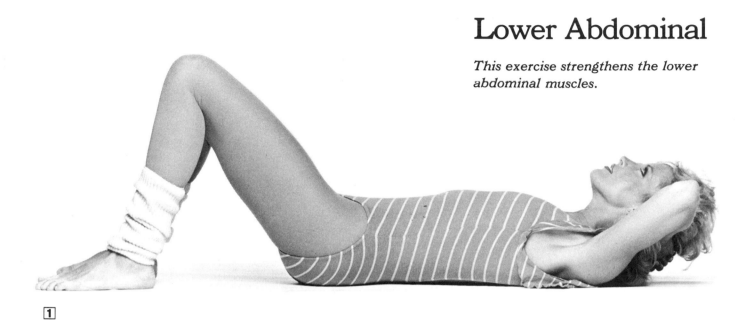

1

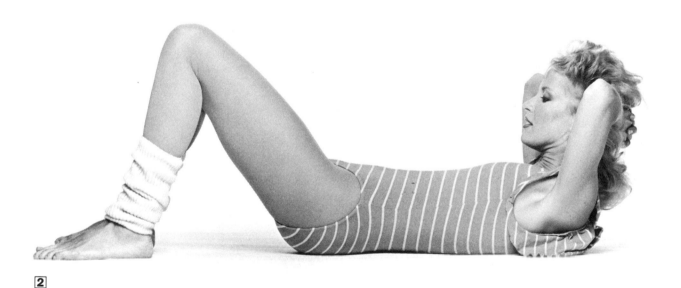

2

1 Lie on your back with your knees raised and close together and your feet flat on the floor. Clasp your hands behind your head, raised slightly from the floor.

2 Keeping your arms at the back of your head, but *not* using their power, lift your head and upper back, with chin up.

Repeat.

Abdominal Release

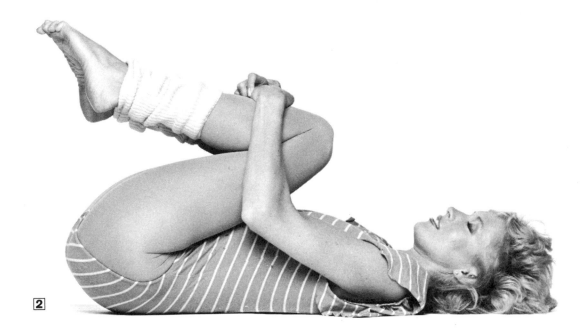

1 Lie flat on your back.

2 Clasp your knees and pull them to your chest. Hold until your abdominal muscles are fully relaxed.

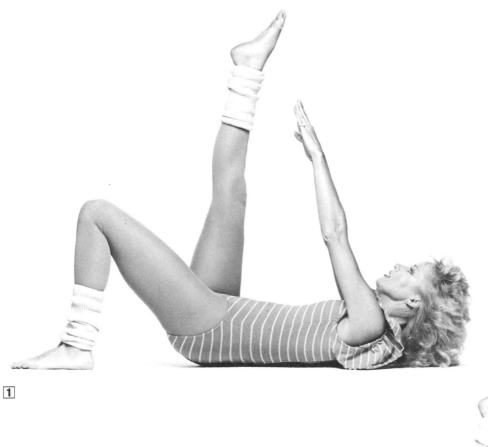

1 Lie flat on your back, with your left knee bent and your left foot flat on the floor, your right leg straight up, toes pointed. Extend your arms toward your raised right foot.

2 Reach for your toes, raising your upper body from the floor. And again.

3 Repeat, reversing the positions of your legs.

REPEAT ABDOMINAL RELEASE

79

Bicycle

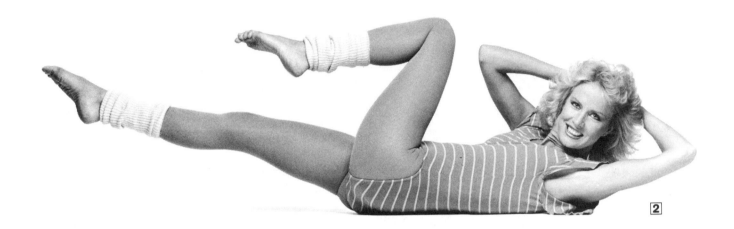

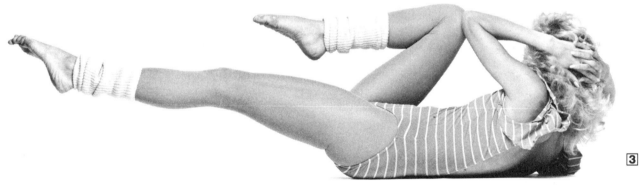

1 Lie on your back, legs out straight, toes pointed. Clasp your hands behind your head, raised slightly from the floor.

2 Raise your legs slightly from the floor. Bend your left leg and draw the knee up toward your chest, reaching for it with your right elbow.

3 Straighten your left leg, keeping it raised from the floor, and draw up your right knee, touching it with your left elbow.

4 Repeat, alternating legs, in a smooth, continuous bicycling motion.

REPEAT ABDOMINAL RELEASE

Dead Cat

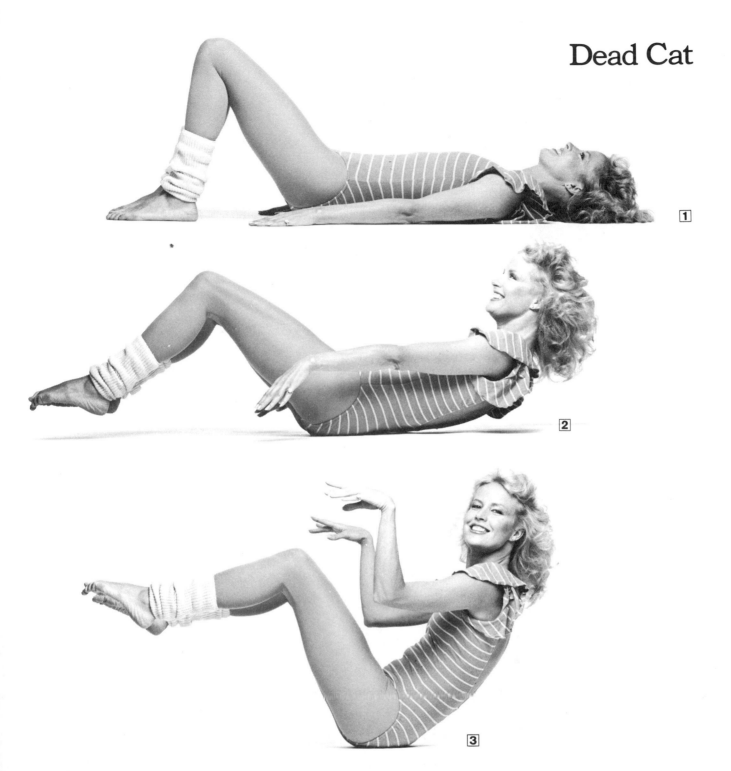

1 Lie on your back with your legs close together, knees bent and feet flat on the floor, and your arms straight alongside your body.

2 Balancing on your buttocks, lift your head, torso, arms, and legs gradually from the floor.

3 Continue lift until you're sitting on the end of your spine, thighs at a 45-degree angle, calves and upper arms parallel with the floor, forearms raised at right angles to upper arms, hands at right angles to wrists, fingers spread.

4 Return to starting position, and repeat.

REPEAT ABDOMINAL RELEASE

Scissors

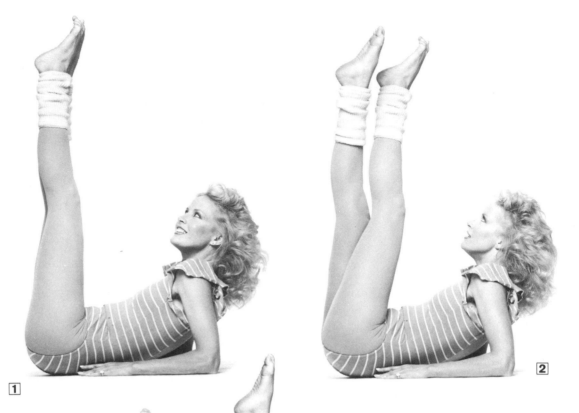

1 Lie on your back, with raised head and shoulders supported by your elbows, forearms at your sides, palms flat on the floor. Lift your legs straight up and point your toes.

2 Cross your left leg over the right, and start to lower them slowly toward the floor.

3 As legs slowly descend, cross your right leg over the left.

4 Keep crossing and re-crossing your legs in a scissors motion until they almost touch the floor. Raise legs, still scissoring, back to your original position.

Repeat.

REPEAT ABDOMINAL RELEASE

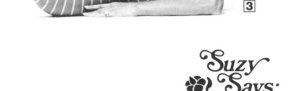

Suzy Says:

"Feel the stretch, then go for more—but not beyond the point where it causes pain. If regular exercise is to be part of your life, it has to fit in comfortably."

Side Stretch

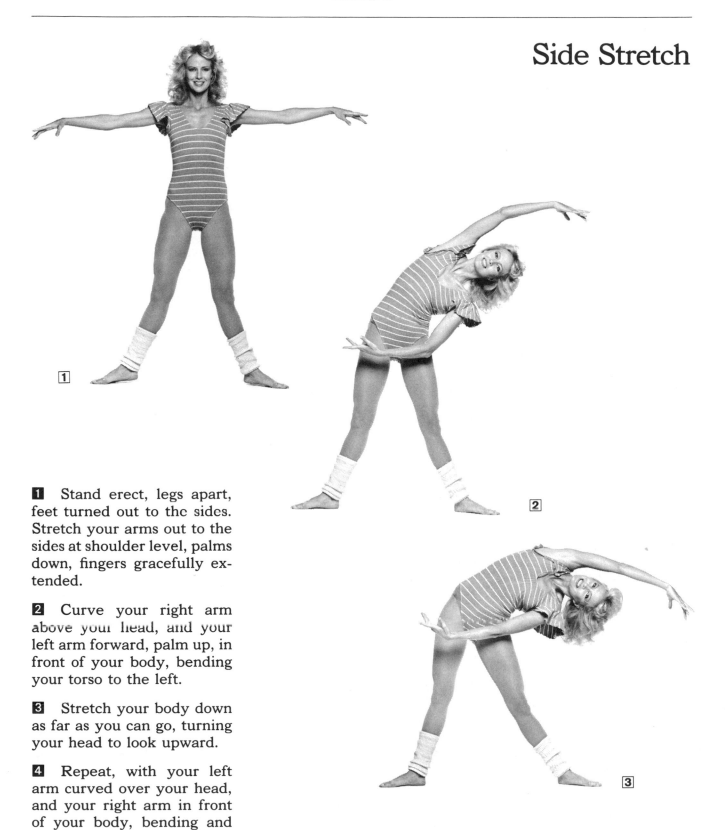

1 Stand erect, legs apart, feet turned out to the sides. Stretch your arms out to the sides at shoulder level, palms down, fingers gracefully extended.

2 Curve your right arm above your head, and your left arm forward, palm up, in front of your body, bending your torso to the left.

3 Stretch your body down as far as you can go, turning your head to look upward.

4 Repeat, with your left arm curved over your head, and your right arm in front of your body, bending and stretching down to the right. Continue, alternating sides.

Stretch Hang

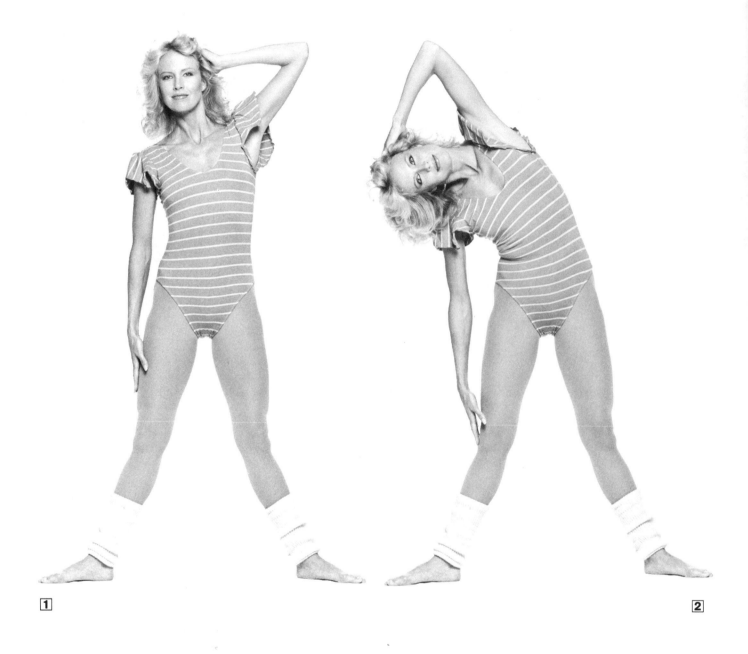

1 Stand erect, legs apart, feet turned out to the sides. Place your left hand on the back of your head, and let your right arm hang straight down, with your hand on your thigh.

2 Bending to the right, stretch your right arm down the side of your leg as far as it will go. Hold for 10 seconds.

3 Reverse the position of your hands and repeat, stretching to the left. Continue, alternating sides.

Waist Swivel

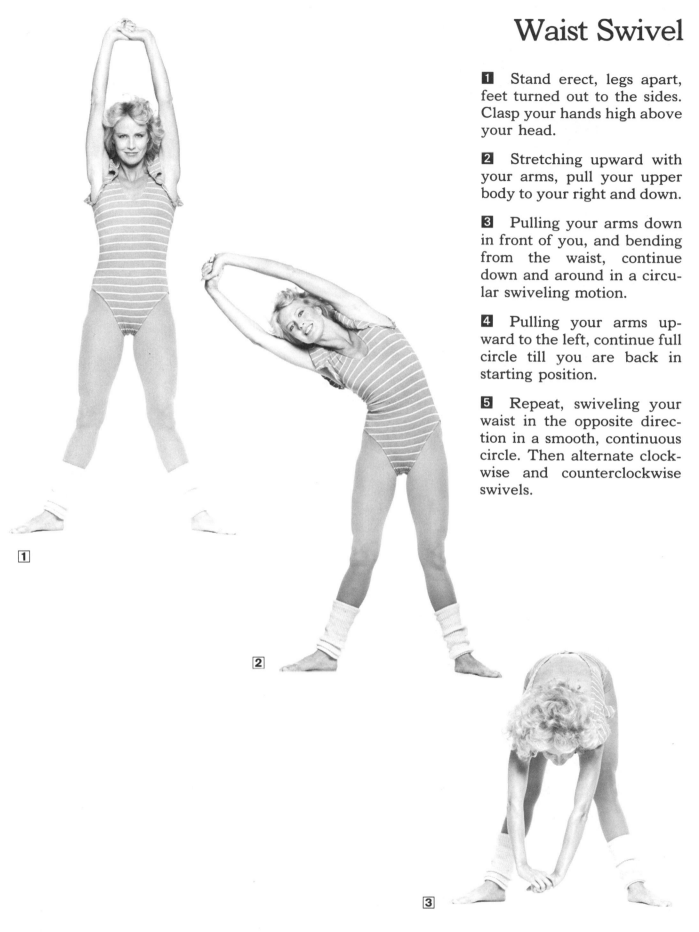

1 Stand erect, legs apart, feet turned out to the sides. Clasp your hands high above your head.

2 Stretching upward with your arms, pull your upper body to your right and down.

3 Pulling your arms down in front of you, and bending from the waist, continue down and around in a circular swiveling motion.

4 Pulling your arms upward to the left, continue full circle till you are back in starting position.

5 Repeat, swiveling your waist in the opposite direction in a smooth, continuous circle. Then alternate clockwise and counterclockwise swivels.

85

Hip Swivel

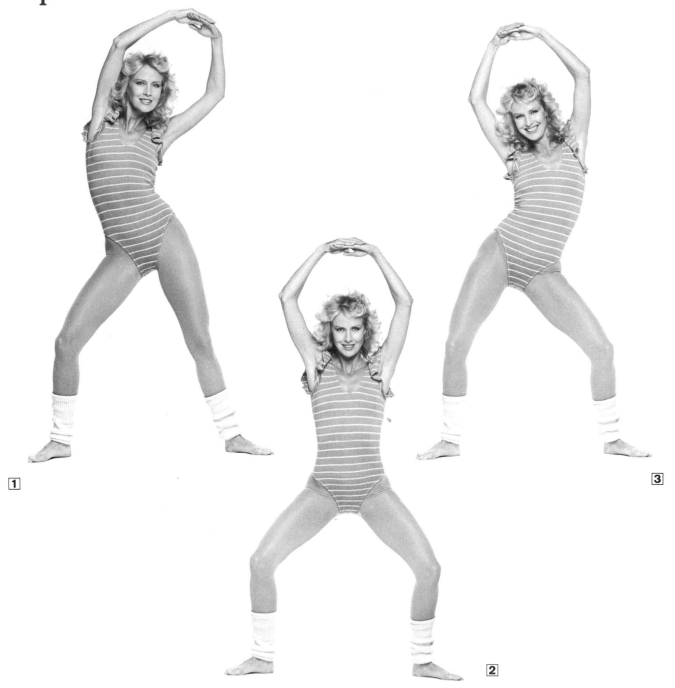

1 Stand with legs apart, feet turned out, and knees always bent. Thrust your hips to the left, at the same time making a left-leaning circle overhead with your arms.

2 Swivel hips to the front, knees bent out to either side, arms directly overhead.

3 Pulling your arms to the right and straightening your right leg, swivel your hips to the right.

4 Continue swiveling motion around to the back, and keep circling.

5 Alternate smooth, continuous circles in clockwise and counterclockwise directions.

Waist-Thigh Stretches

In all spread-eagle positions, knees should face the ceiling to give full stretch to inner thighs.

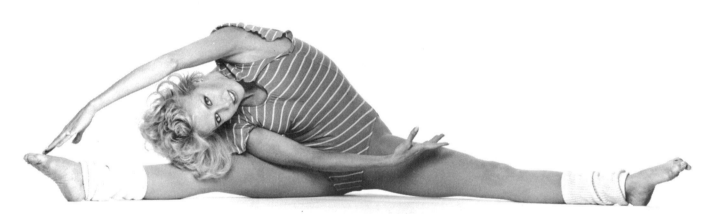

1

2

A.
---

1 Sit on the floor with your legs spread-eagled, your toes pointed. With your right arm curved forward in front of your body, and your left arm curved over your head, bend your torso to the left.

2 Touch the toes of your right foot with the fingers of your left hand.

3 Reverse the position of your arms, and repeat, bending to the right.

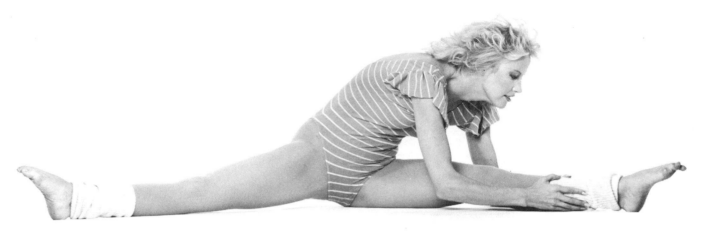

1

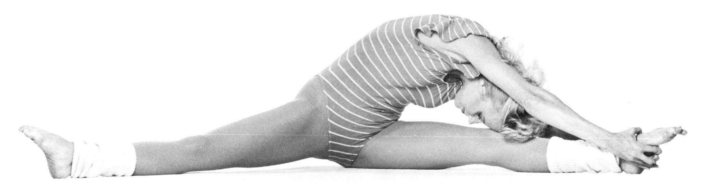

2

B.

1 Sit on the floor with your legs spread-eagled, your toes pointed. Bend forward to the left, and lightly grasp your left leg slightly above the ankle.

2 Pull forward and clasp your hands around your foot, touching your forehead to your left knee.

3 Repeat, bending to your right knee.

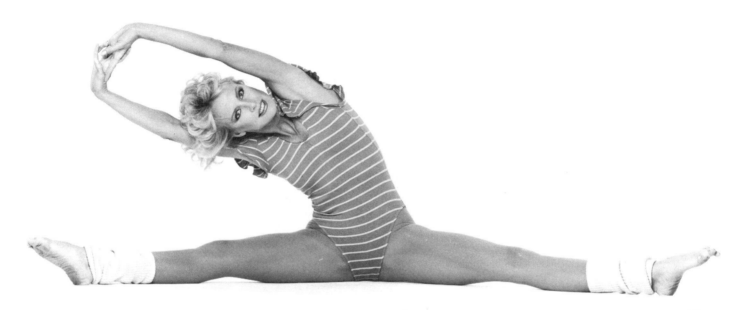

1

C.

1 Sit on the floor with your legs spread-eagled, your toes pointed. Clasp your hands high over your head, and pull your torso to the right.

2 Exerting pull on your arms, stretch as far as you can to the right, then to the left.

3 Repeat, alternating directions.

D.
---

1 Sit on the floor with your legs spread-eagled and your toes pointed. Your hands should be flat on the floor in front of you, almost touching, fingers spread.

2 Bend forward and lightly grasp your ankles.

3 Bending farther forward, stretch your arms wide, touching your feet and aiming for your toes.

Repeat.

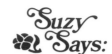

Suzy Says:

"When you exercise, you don't feel like eating so much. You just feel so much better."

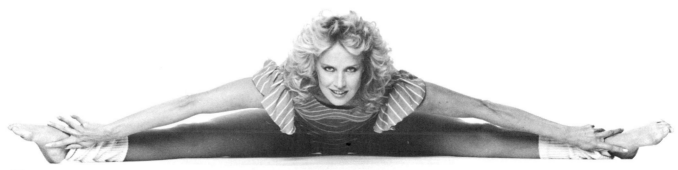

1

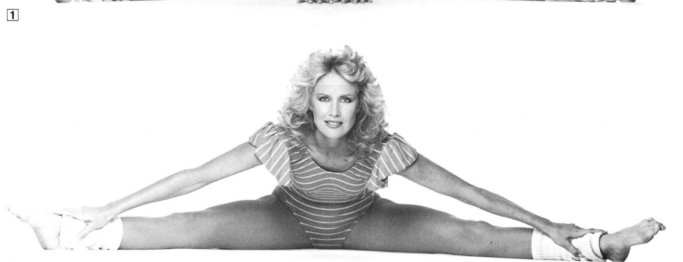

2

3

The Ham Sandwich

This exercise is a hamstring stretch in which the body is folded into a sandwich—hence the title. The hamstrings comprise the muscles in the upper back of the legs.

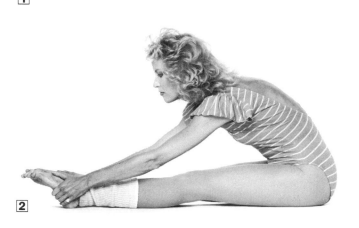

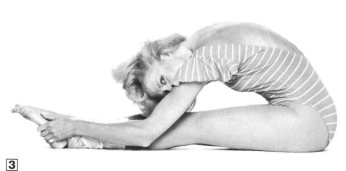

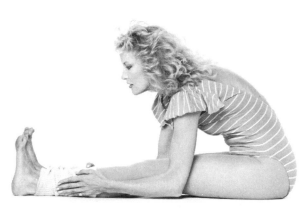

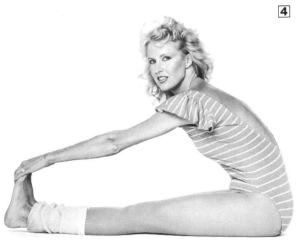

1 Sit on the floor with your legs close together and your toes pointed. Arch your torso forward, and with elbows bent, lightly grasp your ankles.

2 Reach forward, arms extended in a straight line from the shoulders, and grasp the soles of your feet.

3 Bending your elbows and keeping your forearms parallel to your legs, pull your body forward, bowing your head toward your knees.

4 Lift your head and draw your hands back up your legs to mid-calf, elbows bent at a 90-degree angle, and flex your toes upward.

5 Keeping your back as straight as you can, grasp your flexed toes.

Repeat.

Butt Lift

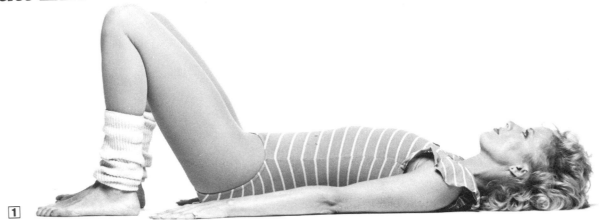

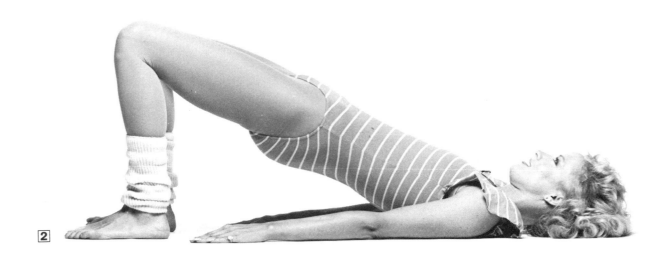

1 Lie on your back with your arms close to your sides, palms flat on floor. Your legs should be about hip-width apart, knees bent up at right angles to the floor, soles flat on the floor, feet pointing straight ahead.

2 Squeezing the muscles of your buttocks as tight as you can, lift your butt until your thighs and torso form an inclined straight line.

Repeat.

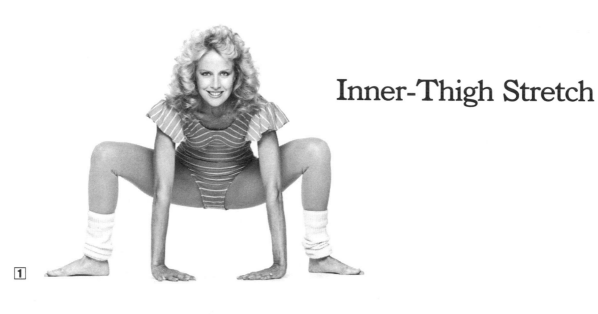

Inner-Thigh Stretch

1

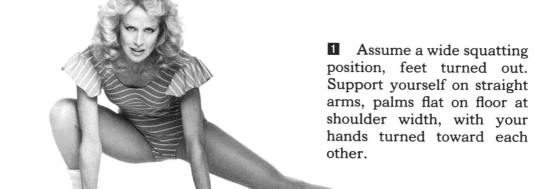

2

1 Assume a wide squatting position, feet turned out. Support yourself on straight arms, palms flat on floor at shoulder width, with your hands turned toward each other.

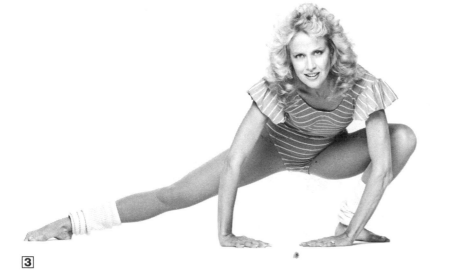

3

2 Shift your weight over onto your right leg, so that your left leg straightens out.

3 Return to starting position, shifting your weight to center. Then shift your weight onto your left leg, so that your step 2 position is reversed.

4 Repeat, alternating left and right leg stretches.

Rovers

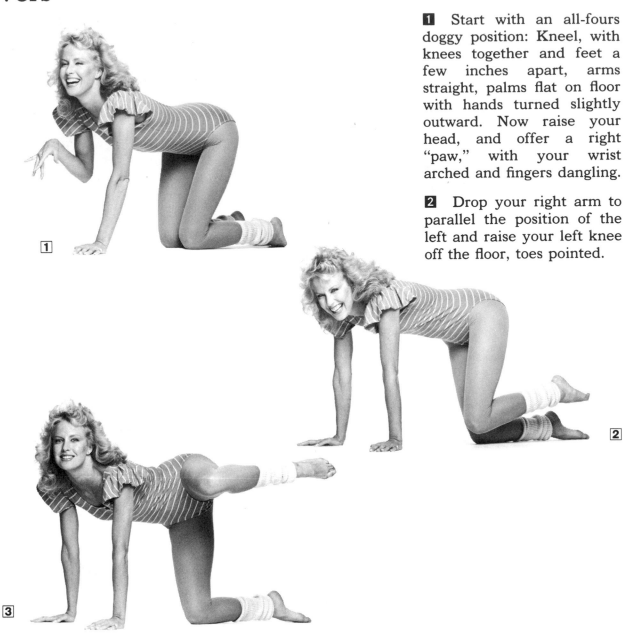

1 Start with an all-fours doggy position: Kneel, with knees together and feet a few inches apart, arms straight, palms flat on floor with hands turned slightly outward. Now raise your head, and offer a right "paw," with your wrist arched and fingers dangling.

2 Drop your right arm to parallel the position of the left and raise your left knee off the floor, toes pointed.

3 Raise your left leg to hip height, parallel to the floor, thigh at right angles to hip, knee bent at right angles to thigh.

4 Repeat steps 2 and 3, this time lifting your left leg as high as you can. Do it several times.

5 Return to starting position and repeat exercise with your right leg.

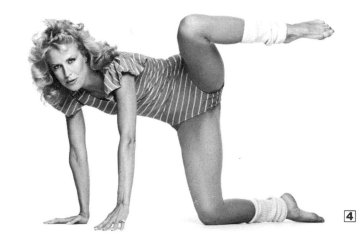

Backside Rovers

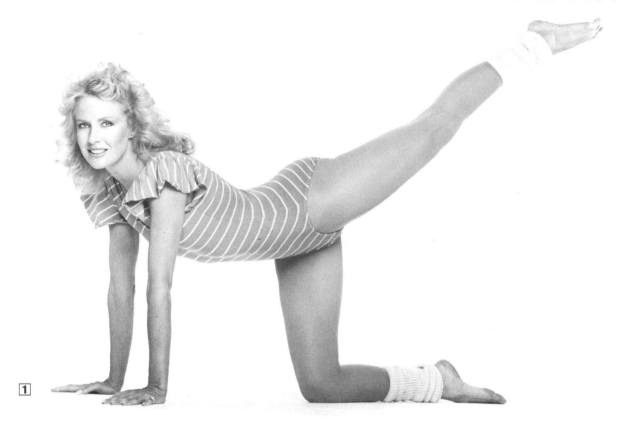

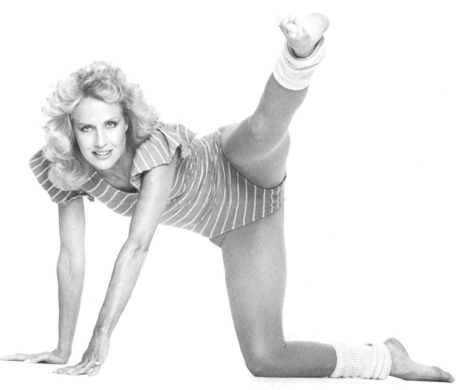

1 Start on all fours, knees together, arms straight and palms flat on the floor with hands turned slightly outward. With head held high, stretch your left leg back and up at a 45-degree angle, toes pointed.

2 Stretch your left leg to the side, at right angles to body.

3 Repeat steps 1 and 2 several times.

4 Return to starting position, and repeat the exercise lifting your right leg.

Elbow Scorpion

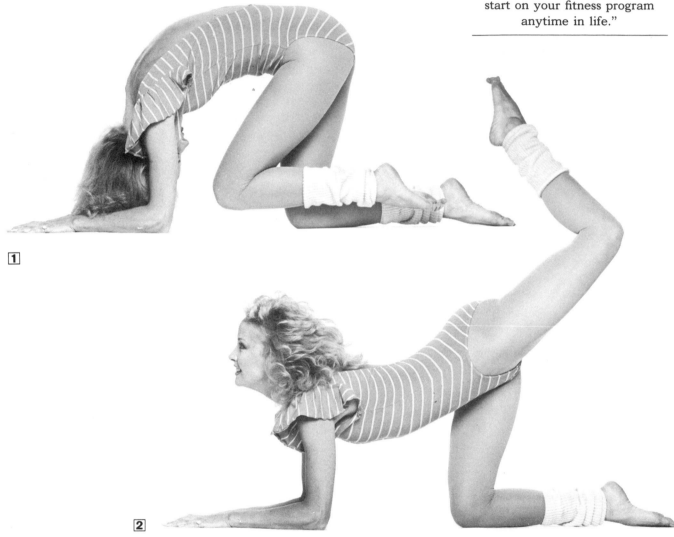

1 Kneel and bend forward, supporting yourself on your elbows, with your forearms straight ahead and your palms flat on the floor. Let your head hang down between your arms, almost touching the floor. Now raise your left knee slightly up and forward.

2 Lift your head as high as you can, while you thrust your left leg—knee still bent, toes pointed—back and up as high as you can.

3 Return to starting position and repeat several times. Then try it with your right leg.

Side Lifts

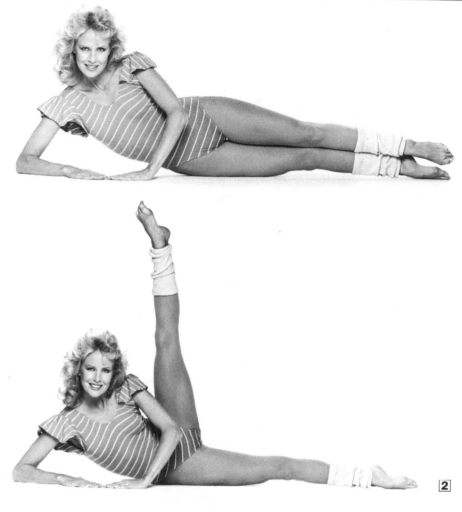

1 Lie on your right hip, legs straight and together, and support your slightly raised torso on your right elbow and forearm. Both palms should be flat on the floor, fingertips touching.

2 Pointing the toes, lift your left leg high, at right angles to the floor.

3 Return to starting position, flex toes, bending up at ankle, and repeat step 2.

4 Starting on left hip, repeat steps 1 and 2 with right leg; then alternate flexing and pointing your foot.

2

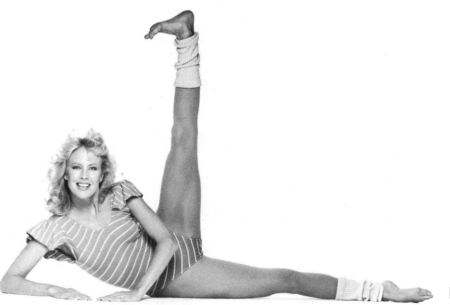

3

Back Leg Lifts

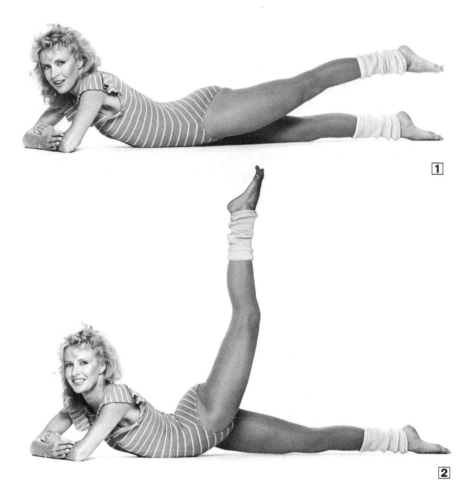

1

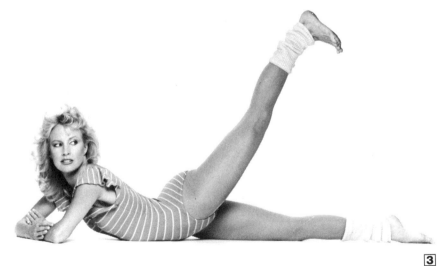

2

1 Lie on your stomach, supporting your raised upper body on your crossed forearms. Raise your left leg slightly from the floor, knee straight, toes pointed.

2 Lift your left leg as high as you can, keeping the knee straight.

3 Return to starting position and repeat step 2, this time with foot flexed, and continue, alternately flexing and pointing your foot.

4 Repeat exercise with right leg.

3

Sagittarian Stretch

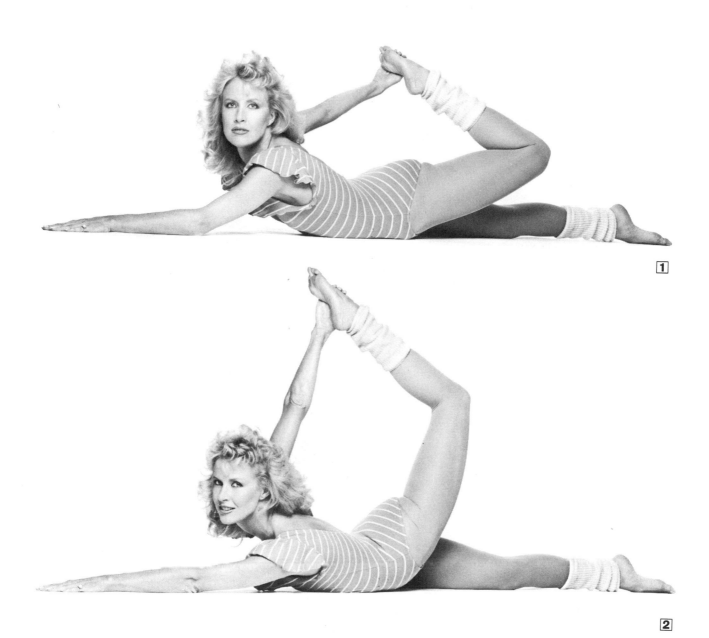

1 Lie on your stomach, head up, torso raised slightly and your left arm extended ahead, palm flat on floor. Bend your left leg up and grasp your left foot with your right hand.

2 Pull your left leg up as high as you can, straightening your right arm.

3 Repeat exercise, grasping your right foot with your left hand; then alternate.

Crossovers

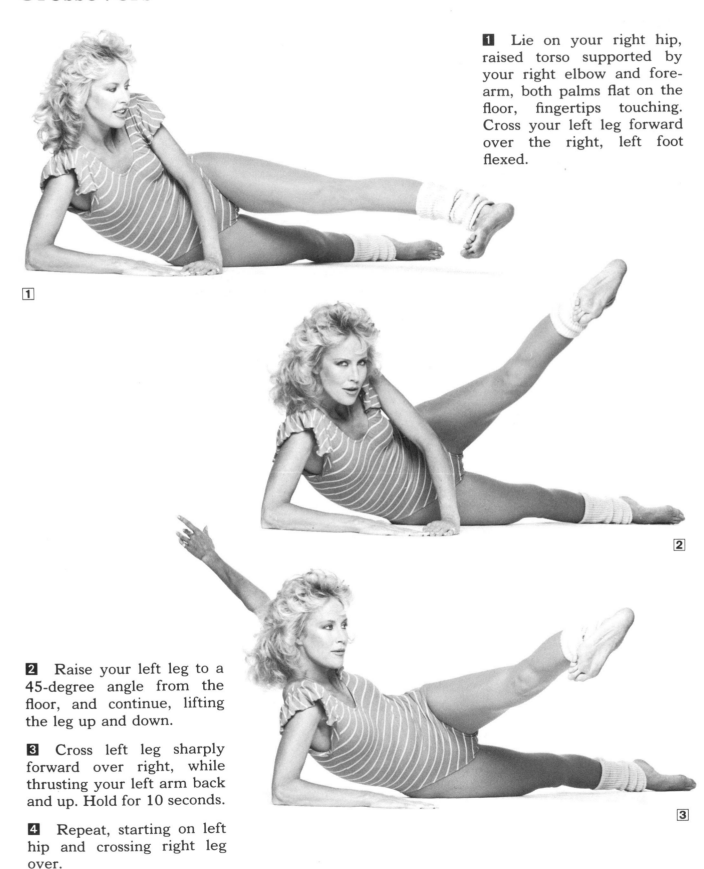

1 Lie on your right hip, raised torso supported by your right elbow and forearm, both palms flat on the floor, fingertips touching. Cross your left leg forward over the right, left foot flexed.

2 Raise your left leg to a 45-degree angle from the floor, and continue, lifting the leg up and down.

3 Cross left leg sharply forward over right, while thrusting your left arm back and up. Hold for 10 seconds.

4 Repeat, starting on left hip and crossing right leg over.

Squat and Waist Stretch

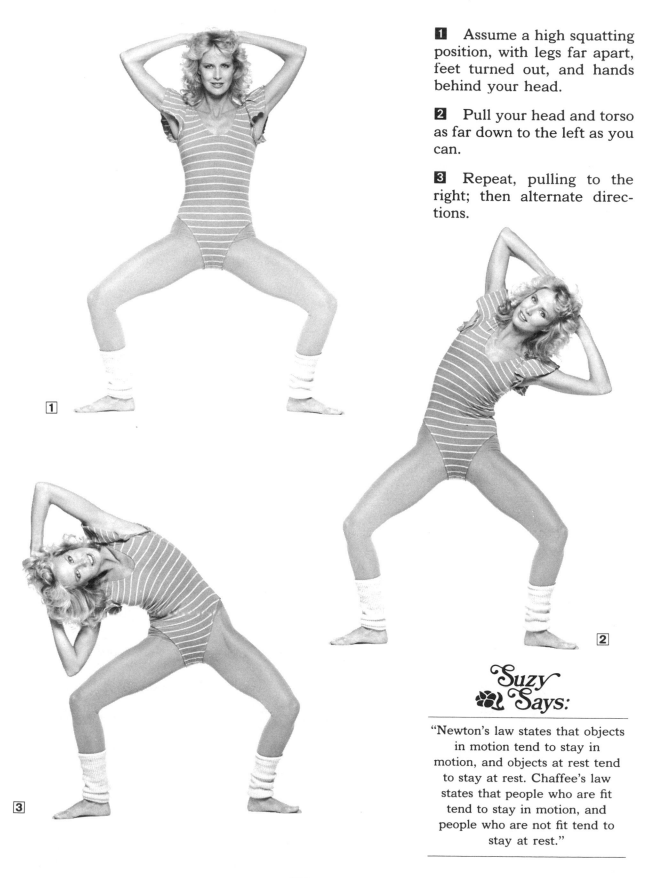

1 Assume a high squatting position, with legs far apart, feet turned out, and hands behind your head.

2 Pull your head and torso as far down to the left as you can.

3 Repeat, pulling to the right; then alternate directions.

Suzy Says:

"Newton's law states that objects in motion tend to stay in motion, and objects at rest tend to stay at rest. Chaffee's law states that people who are fit tend to stay in motion, and people who are not fit tend to stay at rest."

TLC Sit-Up

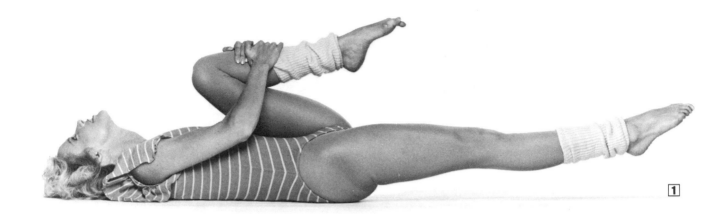

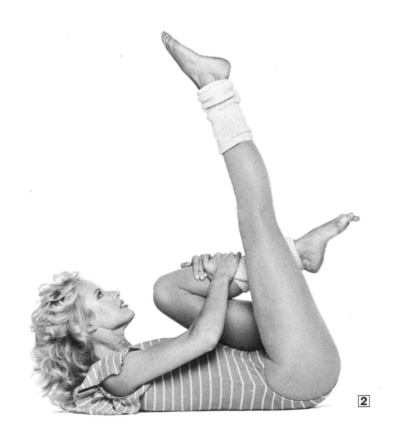

1 Lie flat on the floor, legs out straight, toes pointed. Raising your legs slightly, bend your left knee up and clasp your left leg just below the knee with both hands, pulling it toward your chest.

2 Lift your head as far off the floor as you can while you raise your right leg straight up and as far toward your head as possible. And again.

3 Repeat, reversing the position of your legs.

The Cobra

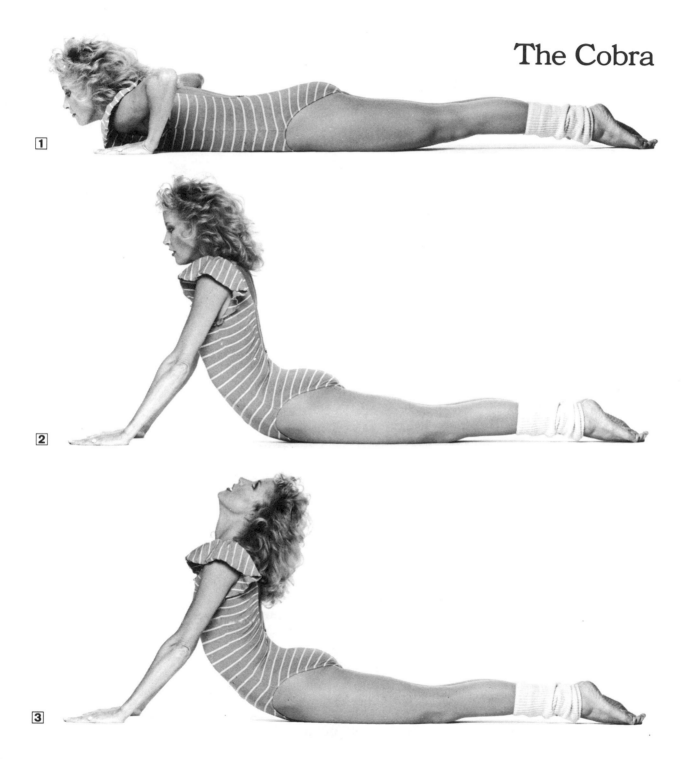

1 Lie on your stomach, legs straight and together, elbows bent up to the sides, hands straight ahead and palms flat on the floor at shoulder level.

2 Straighten your arms, lifting your torso and slowly arching your back.

3 Lean your head back and circle it clockwise and counterclockwise.

Repeat.

The Cross Crawl

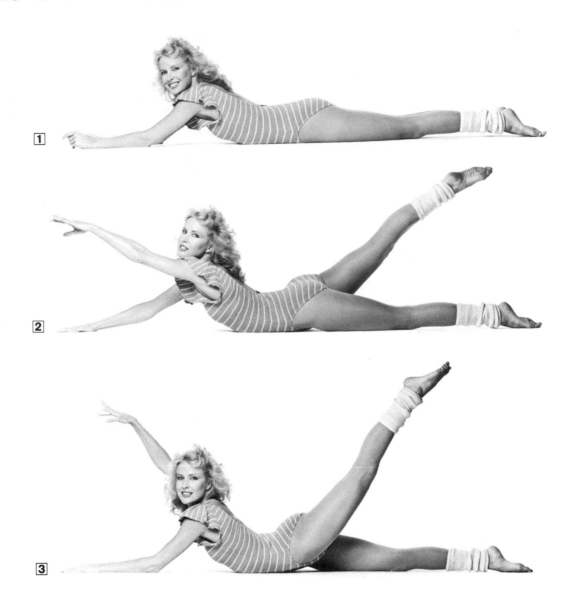

1 Lie on your stomach with your legs out straight and together, your upper body raised, and your forearms extended well out on the floor in front of you.

2 Simultaneously stretch your left arm and your right leg up at an angle of about 45 degrees, without bending your knee.

3 Repeat, raising your right arm and left leg; then alternate.

Cat Stretches

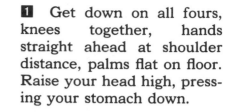

1 Get down on all fours, knees together, hands straight ahead at shoulder distance, palms flat on floor. Raise your head high, pressing your stomach down.

2 Drop your head between your arms. Pressing down on the floor with your hands, pull in your stomach and arch your back up.

Repeat.

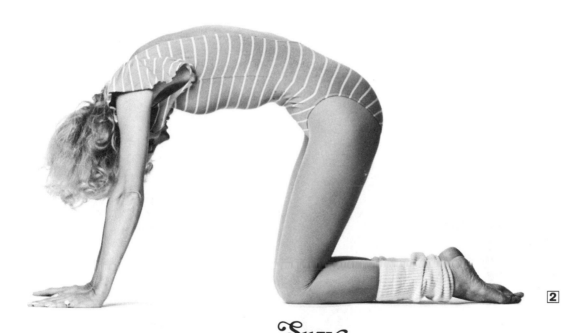

1

2

Suzy Says:

"When you don't exercise, you tire easily. And when you tire easily, you throw away time in which to do so many wonderful things. How much more you can get out of life when you exercise!"

Low Leg Holds

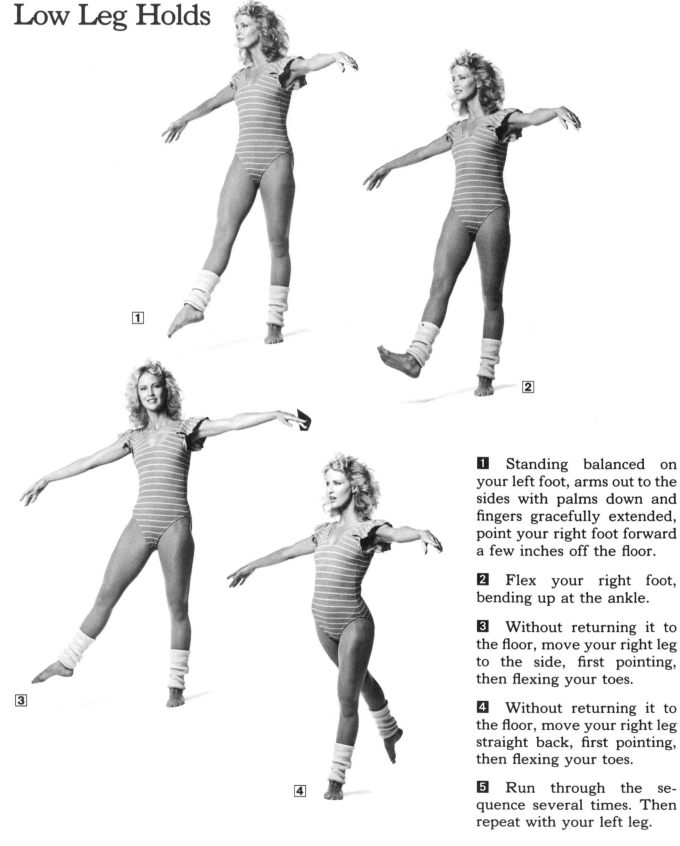

1 Standing balanced on your left foot, arms out to the sides with palms down and fingers gracefully extended, point your right foot forward a few inches off the floor.

2 Flex your right foot, bending up at the ankle.

3 Without returning it to the floor, move your right leg to the side, first pointing, then flexing your toes.

4 Without returning it to the floor, move your right leg straight back, first pointing, then flexing your toes.

5 Run through the sequence several times. Then repeat with your left leg.

Ballet Toe-Ups

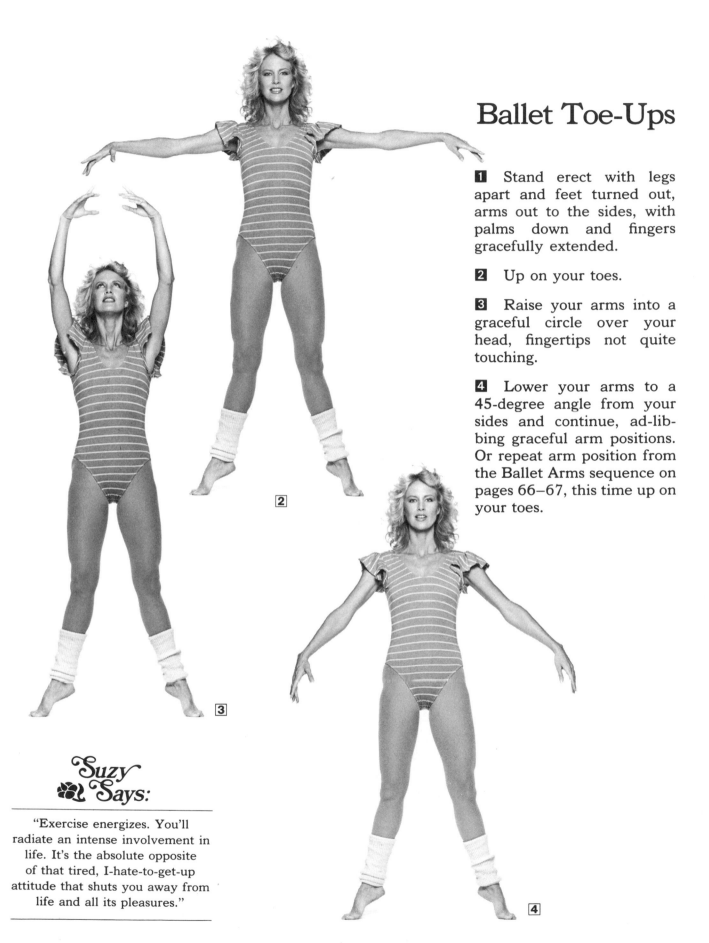

1 Stand erect with legs apart and feet turned out, arms out to the sides, with palms down and fingers gracefully extended.

2 Up on your toes.

3 Raise your arms into a graceful circle over your head, fingertips not quite touching.

4 Lower your arms to a 45-degree angle from your sides and continue, ad-libbing graceful arm positions. Or repeat arm position from the Ballet Arms sequence on pages 66–67, this time up on your toes.

Suzy Says:

"Exercise energizes. You'll radiate an intense involvement in life. It's the absolute opposite of that tired, I-hate-to-get-up attitude that shuts you away from life and all its pleasures."

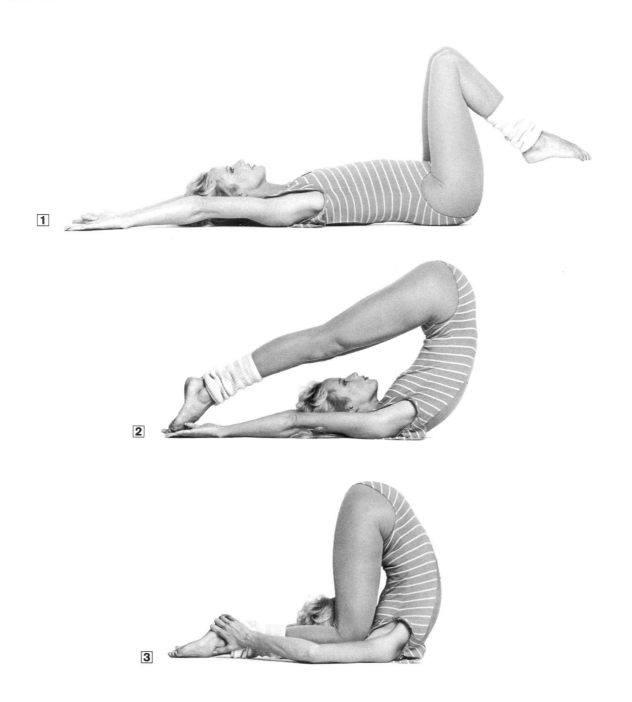

1 Lying on your back, with your arms straight back over your head on the floor, palms up, bend your knees up to form an inverted V. Lift your legs till your thighs are at right angles with your torso, and point your toes.

2 Roll your body slowly up and back over your head, keeping your legs straight, until your toes touch your fingers.

3 Bend your knees to your shoulders, and lightly grasp your heels with your hands.

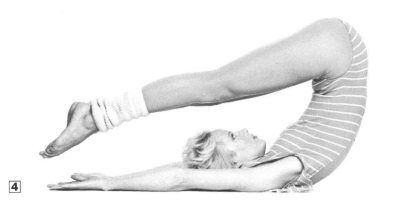

4 Straighten your legs and lift them, keeping knees straight.

5 Raise your legs till your entire body and limbs form a sidewise V, gradually lowering your back to the floor, vertebra by vertebra.

6 Bring your legs on up until they are at right angles to your torso. Then return to starting position.

4

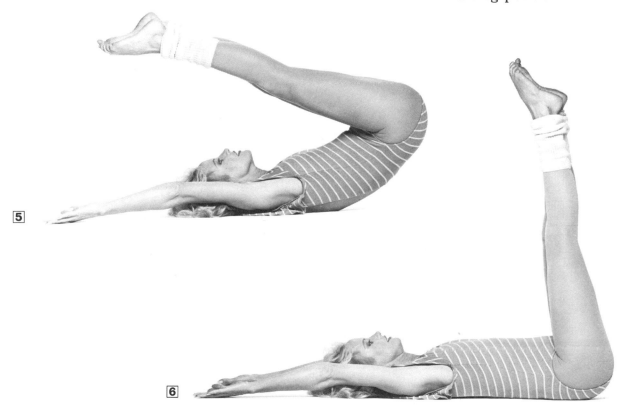

5

6

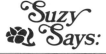

Suzy Says:

"My exercises build all the muscles in your breast area, giving you the best figure you can have without the aid of a bra. If you want that fashionable braless look—exercise."

The Beautiful and Gorgeous Exercises

Beautiful and Gorgeous Exercises are included in the same sequences. Do the Beautiful Exercises first; then, when you've mastered those, add the Gorgeous Exercises to your routine.

In the sequences that include no Gorgeous Exercises, the Beautiful Exercises repeated perfectly will obtain the results of the Gorgeous.

Before starting a Beautiful and Gorgeous Sequence, repeat the corresponding Pretty sequence. For example, do the Pretty Arms sequence as a prelude to the Beautiful and Gorgeous Arms sequence.

Warmups and Cool Off are the same as for Pretty Exercises.

All exercises in this section are Beautiful unless designated Gorgeous.

Underarm Pushups

Repeat Froggy Ups from pages 71–76 until you're strong enough to do a straight body push-up, using the same arm variations and releases. Then give this one a try.

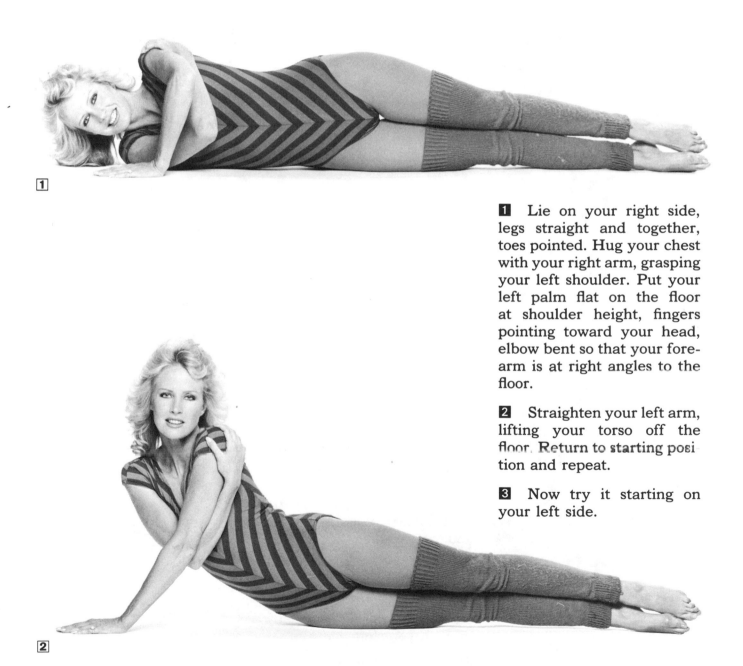

1

2

1 Lie on your right side, legs straight and together, toes pointed. Hug your chest with your right arm, grasping your left shoulder. Put your left palm flat on the floor at shoulder height, fingers pointing toward your head, elbow bent so that your forearm is at right angles to the floor.

2 Straighten your left arm, lifting your torso off the floor. Return to starting position and repeat.

3 Now try it starting on your left side.

Shoulder Stretch

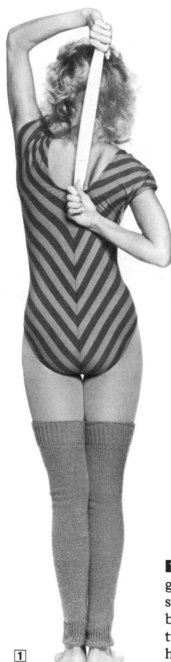

1

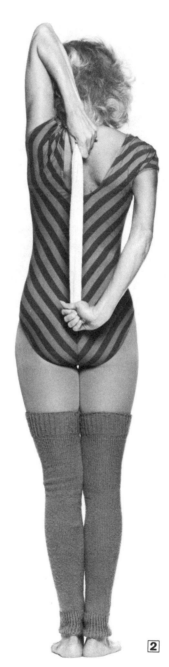

2

1 Stand erect, legs together and feet turned slightly out. Behind your back, hold a ribbon taut between your hands: the left hand just above your head, the right arm bent up behind you to grasp the other end of the ribbon.

2 Keeping the ribbon taut, pull it down with your right hand as far as you can then up with your left.

3 Reverse hands and repeat.

112

Undulations

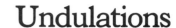

1 Stand with your right leg crossed in front of the left, your feet turned sharply out in opposite directions (as in ballet's fifth position). Curve your right arm down and away from your body, your left arm up and away from your body, palms facing your body, fingers gracefully extended.

2 Raise your right arm and lower the left in undulating, wavelike movements.

3 Reverse the starting positions of your arms and legs, and repeat.

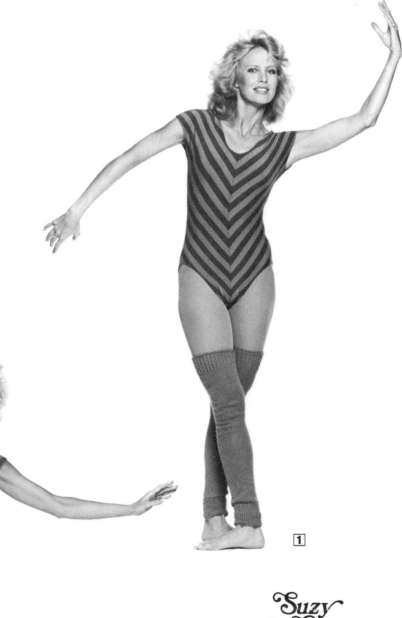

1

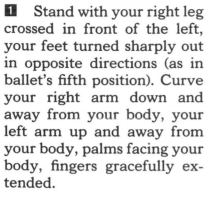

2

Gorgeous Arm Extensions

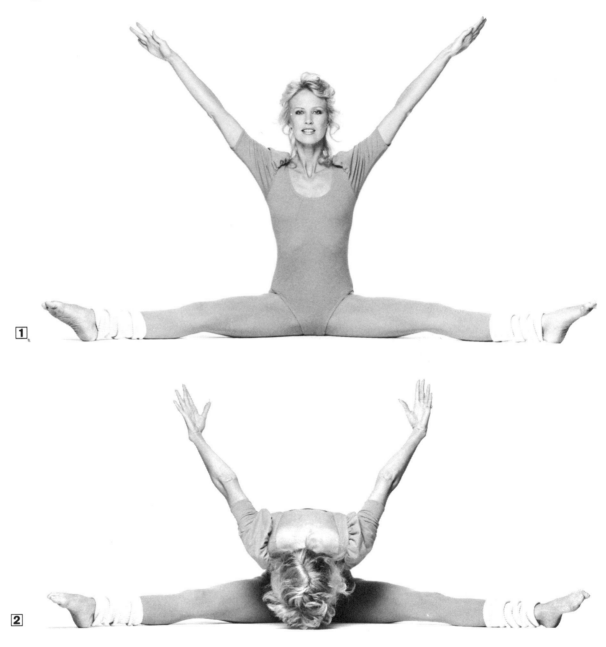

1 Sitting erect, with straight legs spread wide and toes pointed, extend your arms up and out to the sides at a 45-degree angle, palms outward.

2 Roll your torso forward and down until your head touches the floor, your arms flung up behind you, palms facing.

Repeat.

Abdominals

In order to develop your most attractive flat stomach, keep your stomach pulled in as tightly as possible during all the following exercises.

Straight Leg

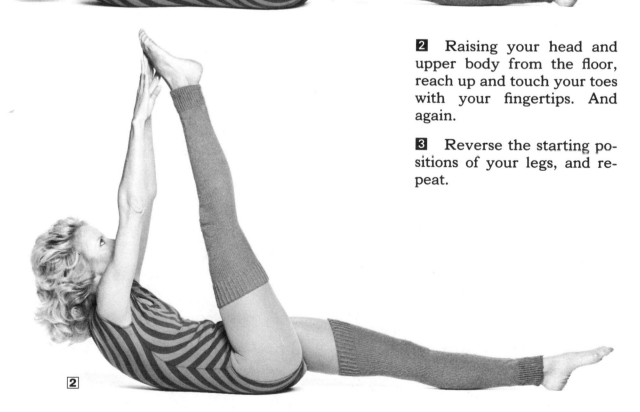

1 Lie on your back, head slightly raised, with your left leg straight, toes pointed, and your right leg straight up at right angles to your body, toes pointed. Raise your arms, hands together, straight toward that right foot.

2 Raising your head and upper body from the floor, reach up and touch your toes with your fingertips. And again.

3 Reverse the starting positions of your legs, and repeat.

115

Release

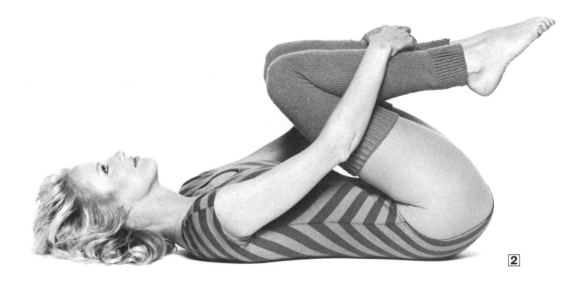

2

1 Lie flat on your back, with your arms straight down at your sides, your legs together, toes pointed.

2 Hug your knees as close to your chest as possible, grasping your legs at mid-calf, and hold position for about 10 seconds.

Tricycle

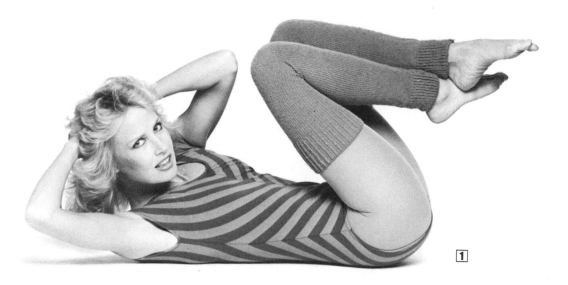

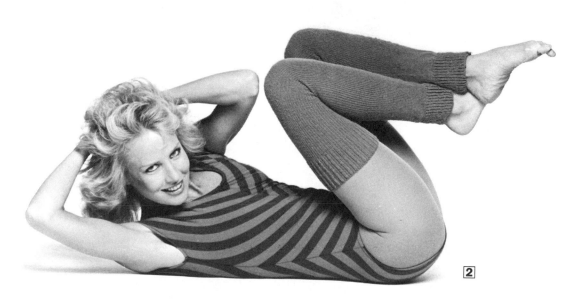

1 Lie on your back, with your knees pulled up toward your chest, left ankle crossed over right, toes pointed. Raise your head slightly, and clasp hands, interlacing the fingers, behind your head.

2 Reach for your right knee with your left elbow.

3 Repeat, with right elbow to left knee; then alternate.

REPEAT RELEASE

Wide Scissors

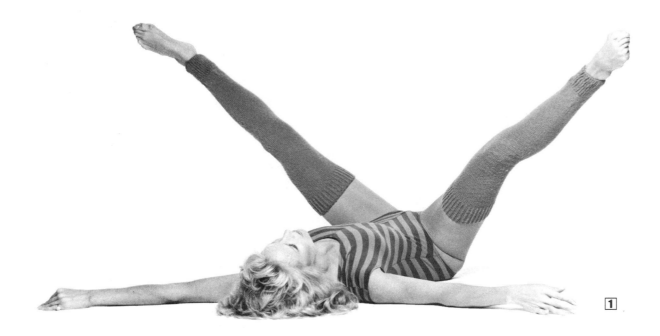

1 Lie on your back, your arms straight out to the sides, your legs raised into the widest possible V, toes pointed.

2 Cross your legs over each other in scissorlike movements while you lower them slowly almost to the floor and raise them back up.

Repeat.

REPEAT RELEASE

Gorgeous Cross-Leg Sit Hold

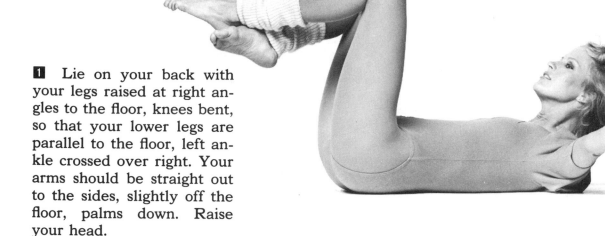

1 Lie on your back with your legs raised at right angles to the floor, knees bent, so that your lower legs are parallel to the floor, left ankle crossed over right. Your arms should be straight out to the sides, slightly off the floor, palms down. Raise your head.

2 Without touching arms or legs to the floor, lift your torso to a sitting position, arching your arms gracefully overhead.

3 Return to starting position and repeat.

REPEAT RELEASE

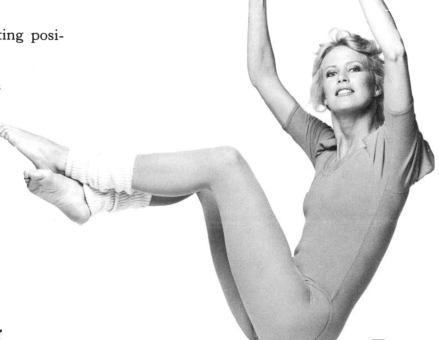

Suzy Says:

"One of the great bonuses of my fitness program is a new enthusiasm for living and loving that the men in your life will find irresistible. I call it emotional sex appeal."

Waist Pulses

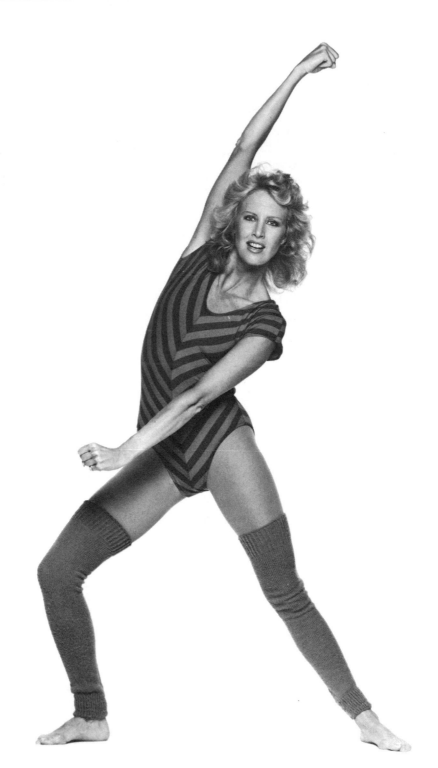

1 Stand erect, with straight legs wide apart and feet turned out, your arms straight down at your sides. Clench your fists.

2 Bending your right knee, thrust your right arm straight up above your head, and your straight left arm diagonally down across your body toward the right knee, stretching your torso in a curve to the left.

3 Reverse the positions of your arms and legs, and repeat; then continue, alternating positions.

Side Swivels

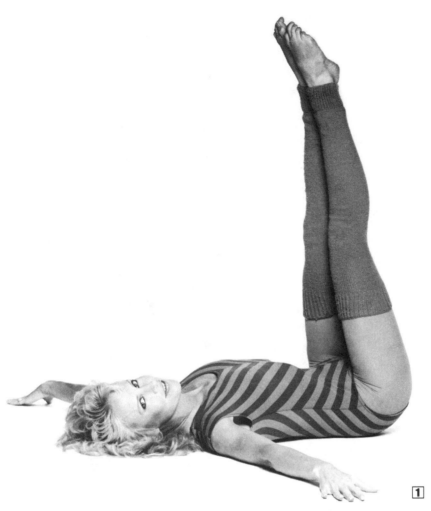

1 Lie on your back, with your arms straight out to the sides, palms down and fingers spread. With knees together, toes pointed, raise your legs straight up at right angles from the floor.

2 Lower your legs as far over to the left as you can without touching the floor.

3 Repeat, swiveling your legs to the right; then alternate.

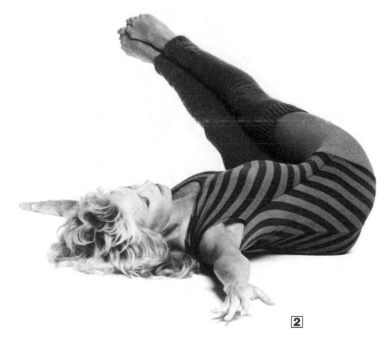

Waist Crunch

1 Kneel, and sit back on your heels, torso and head erect. Clasp your hands behind your head.

2 Bend to the right until your elbow touches the floor.

3 Bend to the left; then alternate.

1

2

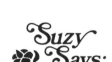
122

Inner Thigh Ups

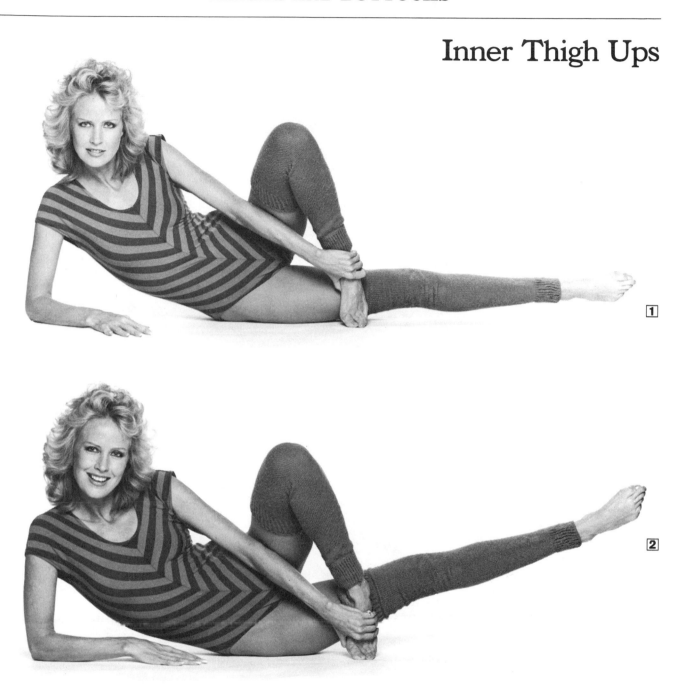

1 Lying on your right hip, support your raised torso on your right elbow, forearm extended flat on the floor parallel to your body, palm down. With your right leg straight out, toes pointed, bend your left leg over the right, placing your toes on the floor in front of your right thigh, the sole resting on the thigh slightly above the knee. Grasp your left ankle in your left hand.

2 Raise your right leg as high as you can. And again.

3 Switch to your left hip and repeat.

Elbow Kicks

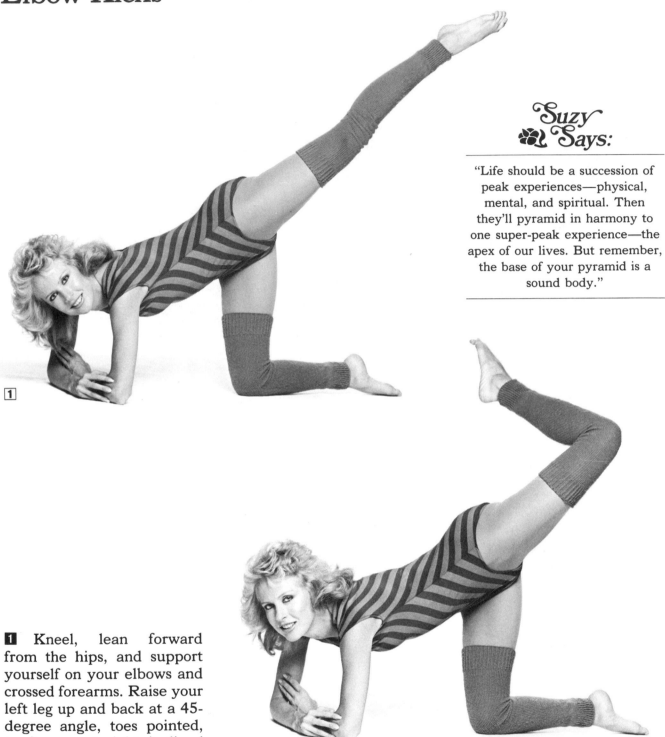

1 Kneel, lean forward from the hips, and support yourself on your elbows and crossed forearms. Raise your left leg up and back at a 45-degree angle, toes pointed, to form a straight inclined line from shoulder to toe.

2 With your knee facing out, bend and straighten your left leg several times.

3 Repeat with your right leg.

124

Doggie Kicks

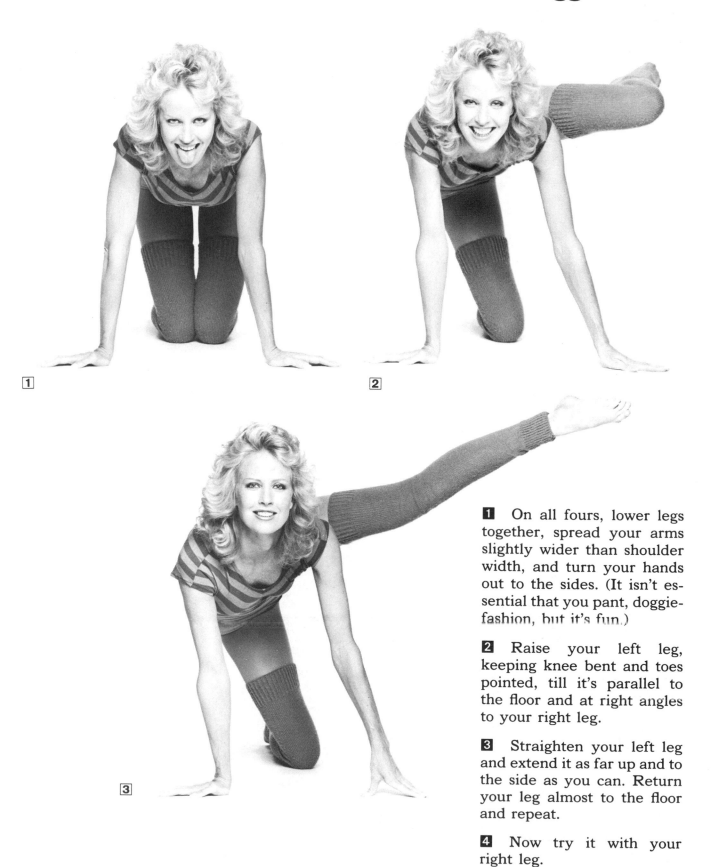

1 On all fours, lower legs together, spread your arms slightly wider than shoulder width, and turn your hands out to the sides. (It isn't essential that you pant, doggie-fashion, but it's fun.)

2 Raise your left leg, keeping knee bent and toes pointed, till it's parallel to the floor and at right angles to your right leg.

3 Straighten your left leg and extend it as far up and to the side as you can. Return your leg almost to the floor and repeat.

4 Now try it with your right leg.

Outrigger

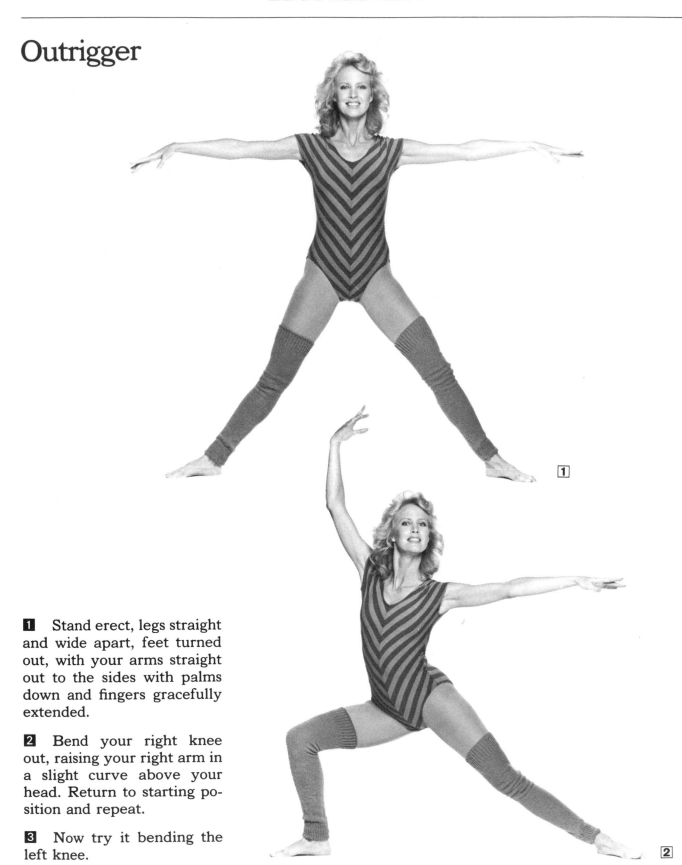

1 Stand erect, legs straight and wide apart, feet turned out, with your arms straight out to the sides with palms down and fingers gracefully extended.

2 Bend your right knee out, raising your right arm in a slight curve above your head. Return to starting position and repeat.

3 Now try it bending the left knee.

Leg Hold

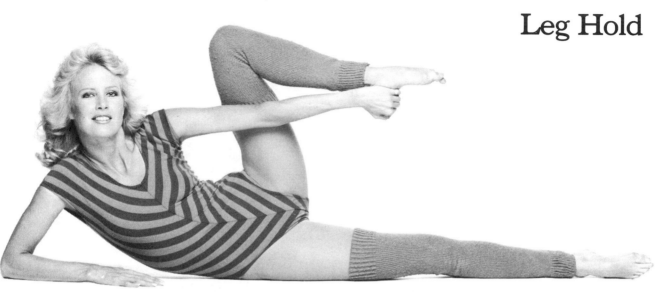

1 Lie on your right side; raise your upper body and support it on your right forearm, placed on the floor parallel to your body, palm flat on the floor, with the elbow slightly above shoulder level. With your right leg out straight, toes pointed, bend your left knee and raise your left leg at right angles to your body. Grasp your left heel in your left hand.

2 Straighten your left leg and bring it back and up toward your head as far as you can.

3 Repeat, starting on your left side; then continue, alternating legs.

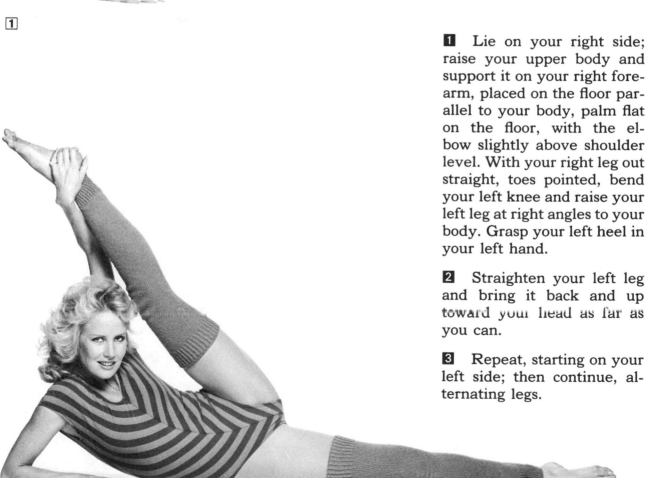

Slalom Jump

For this one you'll need a pillow.

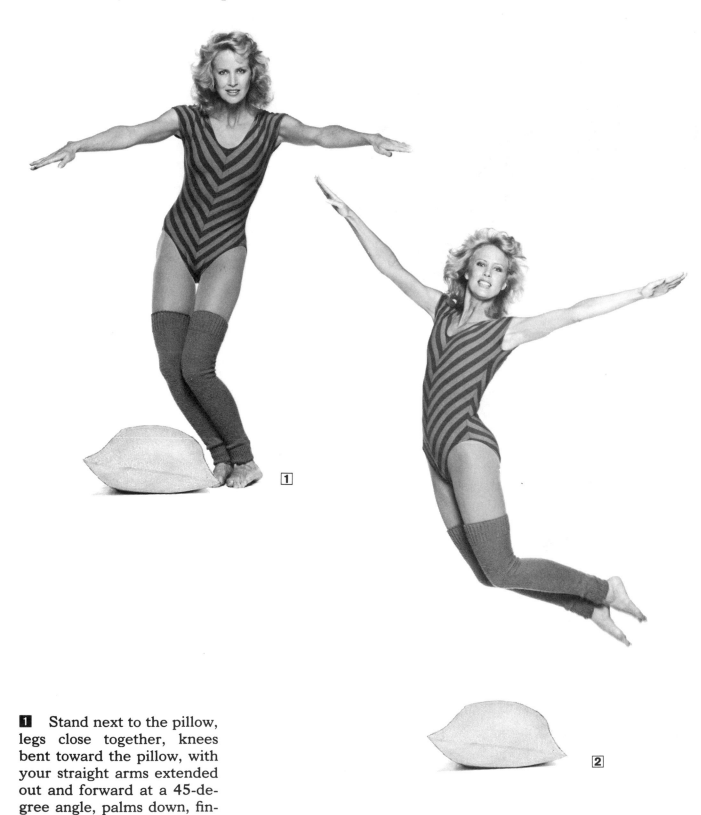

1 Stand next to the pillow, legs close together, knees bent toward the pillow, with your straight arms extended out and forward at a 45-degree angle, palms down, fingers together.

128

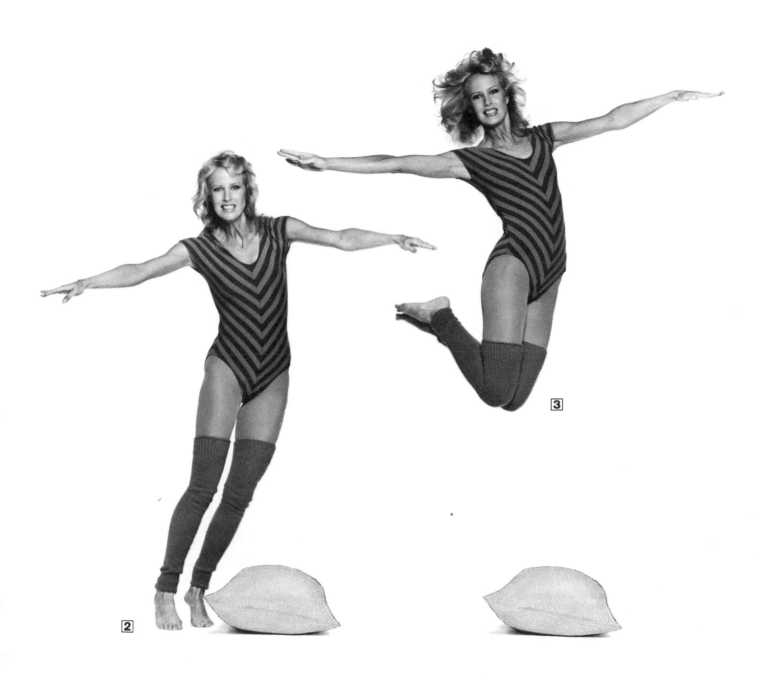

2 Tucking your heels up, jump high across the pillow, landing on the opposite side with your knees bent toward the pillow.

3 Jump back across the pillow in the same fashion, and continue, repeating jumps.

Note: When you first try this exercise, you may add an extra hop on each side until you get the rhythm.

Leg Pull

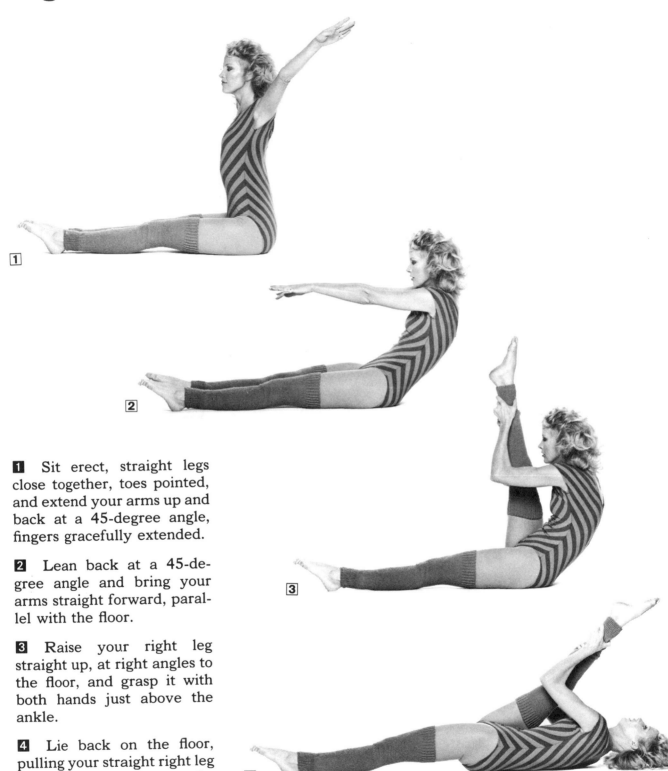

1 Sit erect, straight legs close together, toes pointed, and extend your arms up and back at a 45-degree angle, fingers gracefully extended.

2 Lean back at a 45-degree angle and bring your arms straight forward, parallel with the floor.

3 Raise your right leg straight up, at right angles to the floor, and grasp it with both hands just above the ankle.

4 Lie back on the floor, pulling your straight right leg back toward your head as far as you can.

5 Repeat with your left leg; then continue, alternating legs.

Gorgeous Crab Walk

1 Squat down, with torso erect and feet turned out below wide-spread knees. Your arms should come straight down between your legs, fingertips touching the floor. (From this position I can't resist going into my monkey act.)

2 Walk forward in this position, raising your heels from the floor as you shift your weight from side to side, and helping your balance by touching your fingers to the floor, first right, then left.

3 For release, shake out your legs.

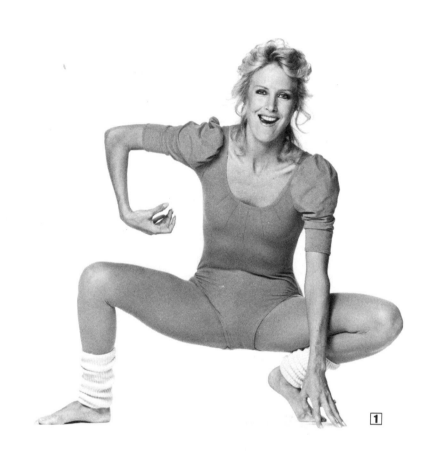

2

1

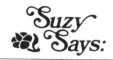

Suzy Says:

"The President's Council on Physical Fitness and Sports reports that a sound program of exercise and nutrition can do more for the health of Americans than all the medicines combined."

Back-Ups

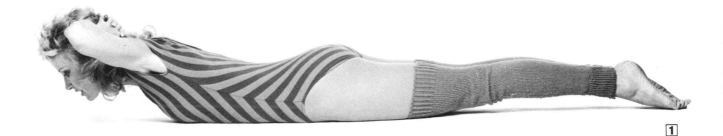

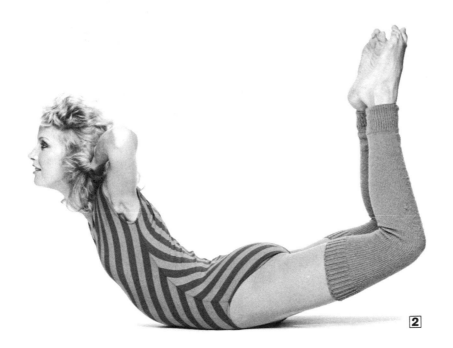

1 Lie face downward, legs out straight and together. Clasp your hands together, interlacing your fingers, behind your head, and raise head slightly from the floor.

2 Arch your back, bend your knees, and reach for the sky with both head and pointed toes.

Repeat.

132

Scorpion

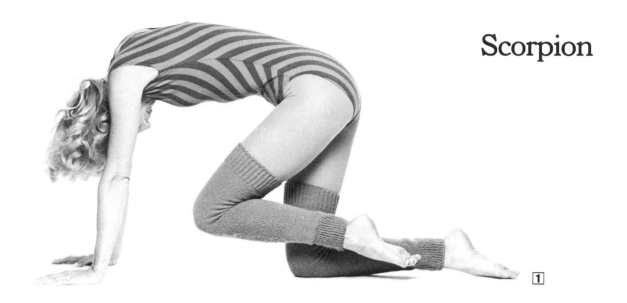

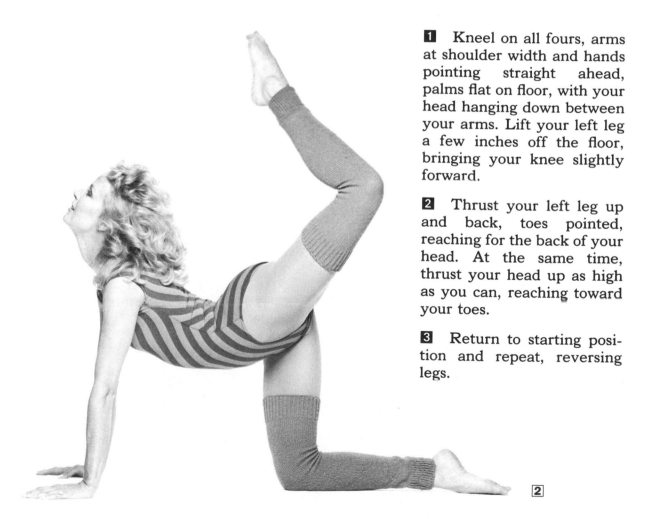

1 Kneel on all fours, arms at shoulder width and hands pointing straight ahead, palms flat on floor, with your head hanging down between your arms. Lift your left leg a few inches off the floor, bringing your knee slightly forward.

2 Thrust your left leg up and back, toes pointed, reaching for the back of your head. At the same time, thrust your head up as high as you can, reaching toward your toes.

3 Return to starting position and repeat, reversing legs.

Gorgeous Front Roll

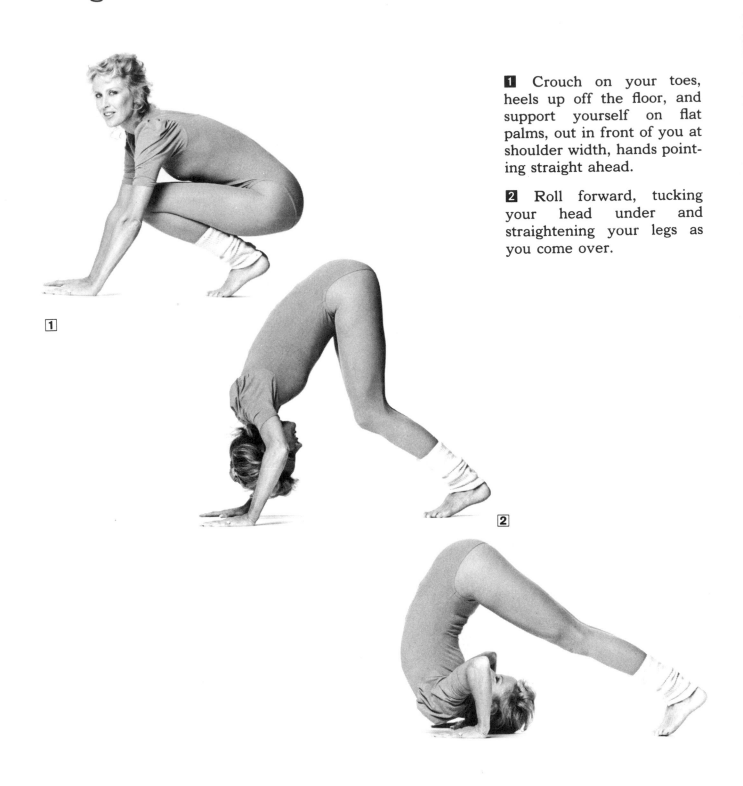

1 Crouch on your toes, heels up off the floor, and support yourself on flat palms, out in front of you at shoulder width, hands pointing straight ahead.

2 Roll forward, tucking your head under and straightening your legs as you come over.

3 As you come over on your shoulders and upper back, point your toes and legs out in a straight line from hip to toe, parallel to the floor.

4 Continue to roll onto your back and up into a crouch, extending your arms out straight before you.

5 Lean forward into starting position, and repeat.

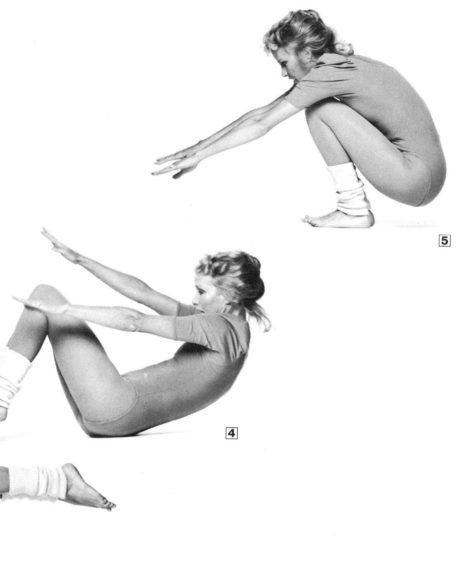

5

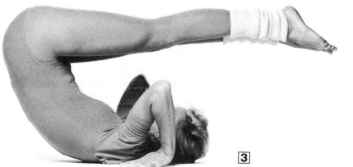

4

3

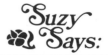

Front High-Leg Balance

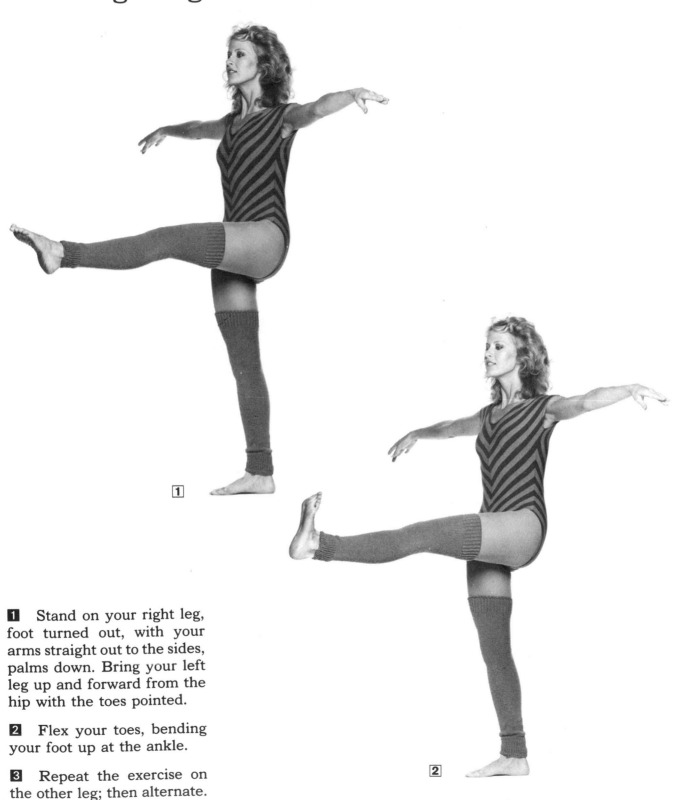

1 Stand on your right leg, foot turned out, with your arms straight out to the sides, palms down. Bring your left leg up and forward from the hip with the toes pointed.

2 Flex your toes, bending your foot up at the ankle.

3 Repeat the exercise on the other leg; then alternate.

Back High-Leg Balance

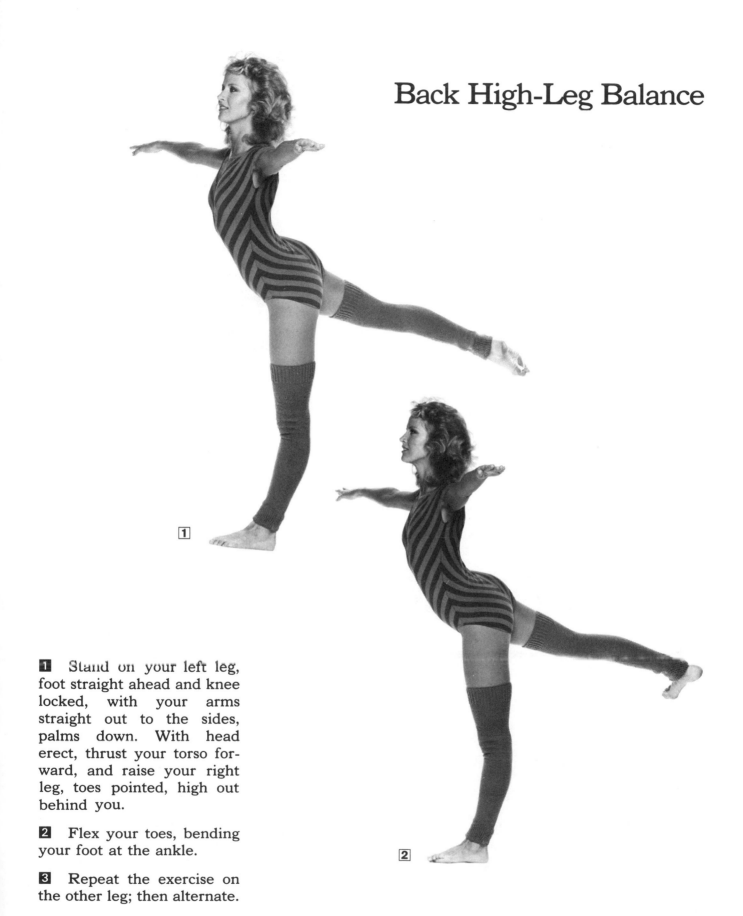

1 Stand on your left leg, foot straight ahead and knee locked, with your arms straight out to the sides, palms down. With head erect, thrust your torso forward, and raise your right leg, toes pointed, high out behind you.

2 Flex your toes, bending your foot at the ankle.

3 Repeat the exercise on the other leg; then alternate.

Front High-Leg Kick

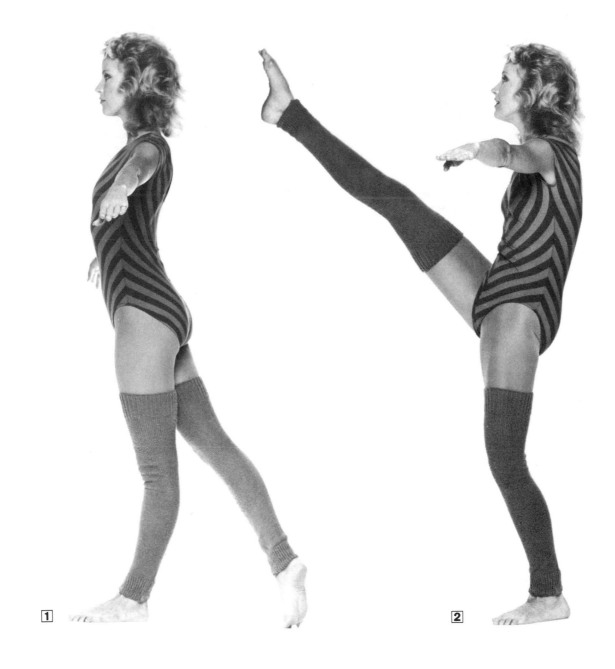

1 Stand on your left leg, foot straight ahead and knee locked, with your arms straight out to the sides, palms down. Place your right leg back, balancing on the tips of the toes, while your torso is thrust slightly forward.

2 Kick your straight right leg forward and up, as high as you can.

3 Repeat, kicking with your left leg; then alternate.

Yoga Balance

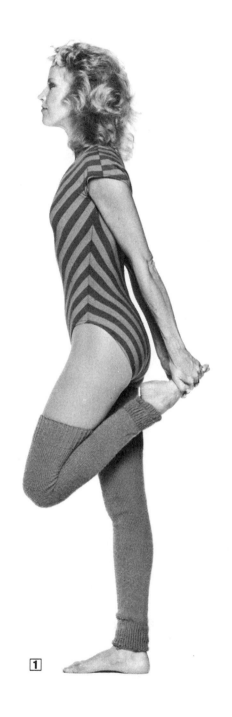

1 Stand on your right leg, foot straight ahead, and fold your left leg up behind you, reaching down behind your back to grasp your left foot, first in your left hand, then in both hands. Hold position for 10 seconds.

2 Repeat, standing on your left foot.

Gorgeous Knee Swivels

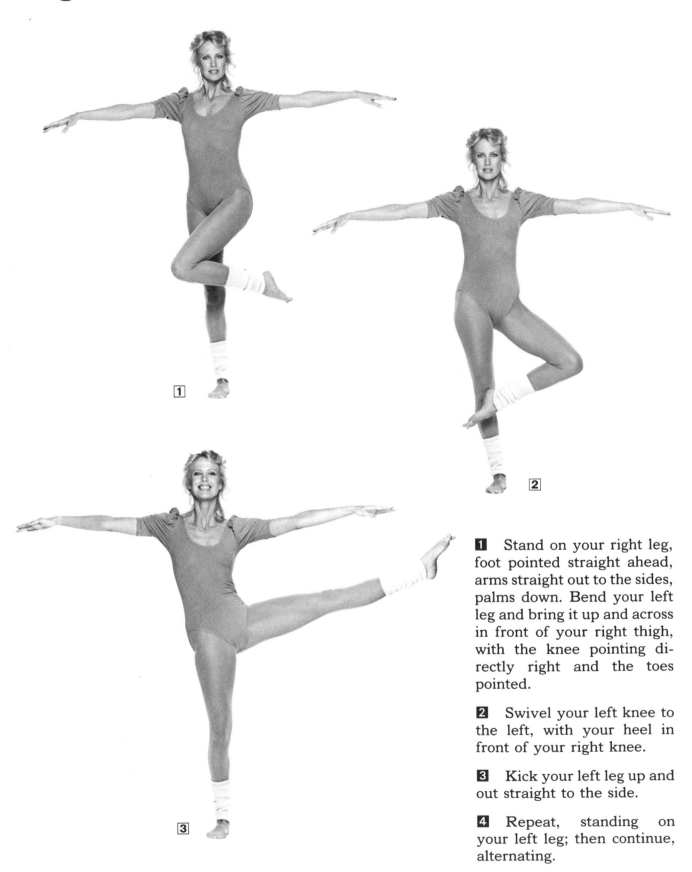

1 Stand on your right leg, foot pointed straight ahead, arms straight out to the sides, palms down. Bend your left leg and bring it up and across in front of your right thigh, with the knee pointing directly right and the toes pointed.

2 Swivel your left knee to the left, with your heel in front of your right knee.

3 Kick your left leg up and out straight to the side.

4 Repeat, standing on your left leg; then continue, alternating.

Anywhere, Anytime

Exercises

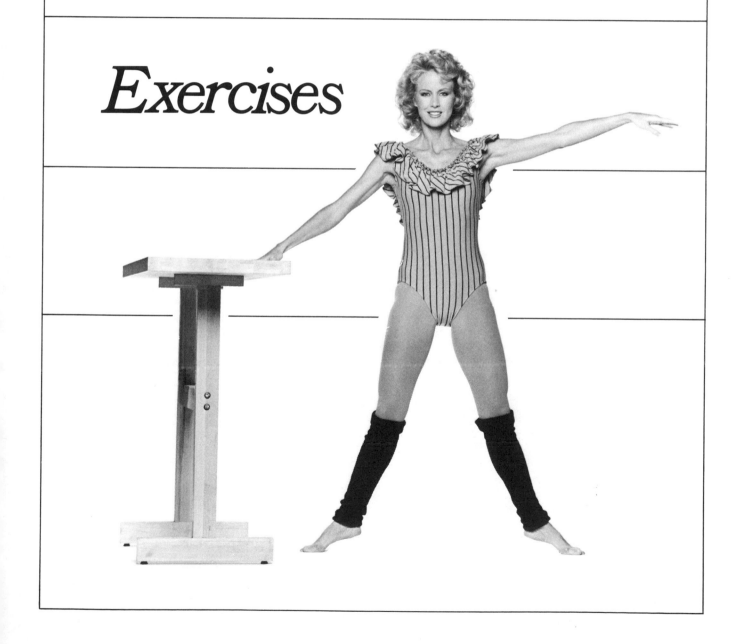

There are days when I do a good half-hour's workout in the morning and catch a ballet class in the afternoon. Those are my ideal days. But New York, New York, that wonderful town, is a time eater, and there are days when I don't have that precious hour. That's why I invented these Anywhere, Anytime Exercises. Do some or all of them when your hectic life takes too big a bite out of *your* time.

Just don't let a day go by without exercise. You *know* what it means to your body, but do you realize it can make your brain cells glow as well? I found out about this the hard way. When my Olympic days were over, my activity level dropped and so did my thinking level. I just had to do something about it, and that's when I helped create free-style ballet skiing, an artistic, expressive form of skiing in which I can stay interested for life. Once I got back into action, I found I could think clearly, sharply, deeply, and quickly again. So remember this: When you exercise, you can use your full brain power.

I've heard some women say, "It's ridiculous doing exercises at bus stops or while I'm working. There are more important things on my mind, and if I can't find the time to exercise, I just won't. All this fuss to look beautiful—it's frivolous!"

This attitude springs from the widespread old belief that beauty is synonymous with low intelligence. What a mistake that is!—our brightest and best men and women in all fields are mainly attractive people.

Just look at my family. Kim graduated *cum laude* from Harvard. Rick has a doctorate in economics. Mark has his master's in physics. Dad is an inventor. My Super-Mom is probably the nation's Number 1 readaholic. And as for me . . .

I never believed a college diploma is a license to stop learning. At UCLA, and the universities of Denver, Washington, and Innsbruck (Austria), I studied everything I thought would be valuable in life: languages, journalism, political science, photography, psychology, and much more. It felt terrific to be power-packed with know-how when I locked horns with some of the toughest opposition in the world in my successful struggle for the Amateur Sports Act of 1978, for Olympic reforms, and for greater government and industry support for national fitness. I fight the good fight with intelligence and know-how. But I fight it better when I add beauty and sex appeal.

No, it's not frivolous to be beautiful. Don't ever stop exercising. If you can't exercise at a regular time in your home or in a gym, keep in the swing with my Anywhere, Anytime Exercises. Don't get in the way of your own greatness. Don't be afraid to be as beautiful as you are.

In Bed

These are exercises to get you going in the morning. But *bed* in the stream of consciousness of most of us eventually leads to *sex*—and what's the relation of fitness to sex?

Fitness does wonders for your love life. According to a study made at the Munich Olympics, more athletes have more sex with more satisfaction than do non-athletes. And that includes women athletes, of course. The fact is, guys' attitudes to muscles have changed. Men appreciate my muscle tone, and they'll appreciate yours. Fitness is sexiness.

Pelvic Lift

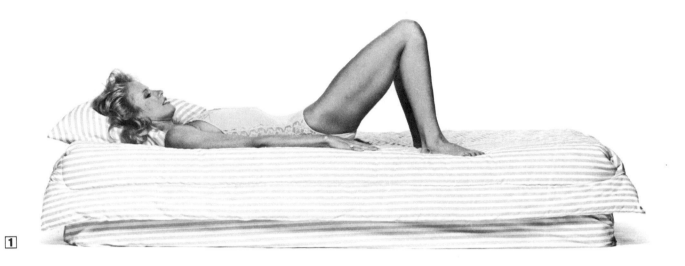

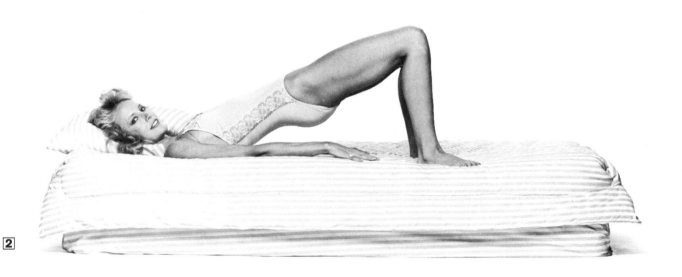

1 Lie with your head on the pillow, knees up a few inches apart, and feet turned slightly out.

2 Raise your hips off the bed, keeping your body in a straight diagonal line from knee to chest and squeezing the muscles of your buttocks tight.

Repeat.

Curl-Up Stretch

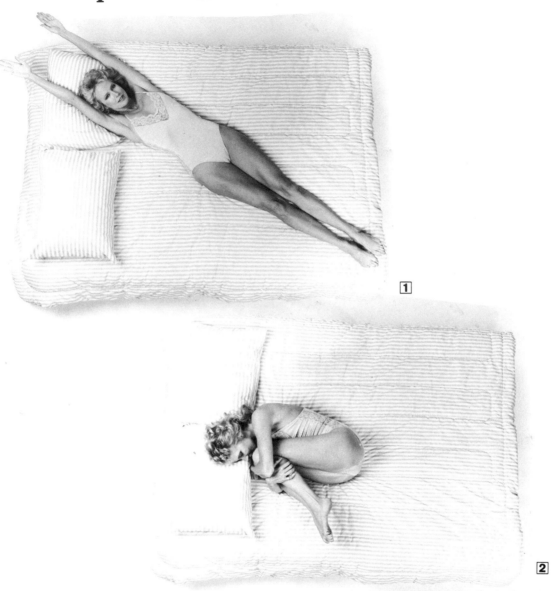

1

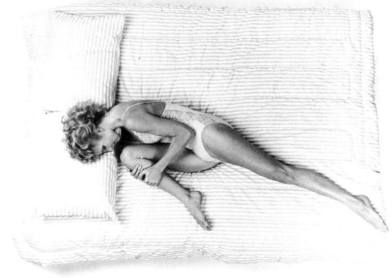

2

3

1 Lie diagonally across the bed, with your legs together and your toes pointed, and stretch your arms over your head, palms upward.

2 Very slowly, breathing deeply, turn onto your right side and hug your knees to your chin with both arms.

3 Extend your left leg out straight, continuing to clasp your right leg in both hands.

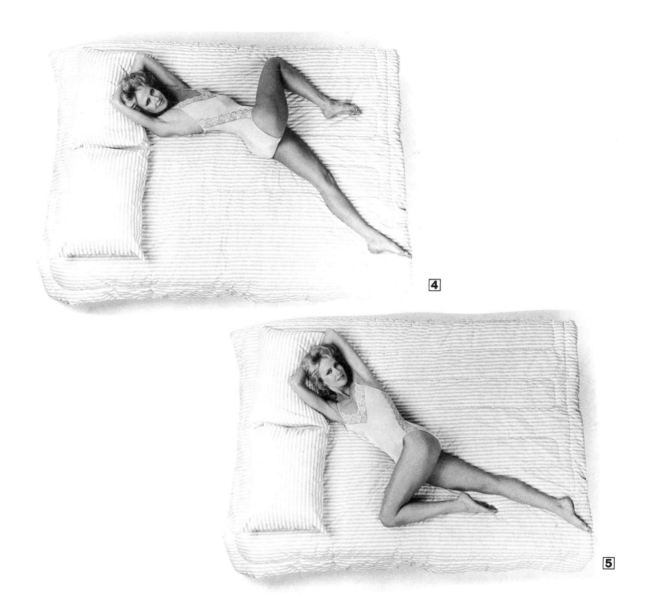

4 Folding your arms behind your head, roll over onto your left side, bringing your bent right leg over the left, and touching the bed with your right knee.

5 Turn back onto your right side and touch your knee to the bed on the right.

6 Return to the starting position and repeat the exercise, this time turning onto your left side; then continue, alternating sides.

Super Waist Crunch

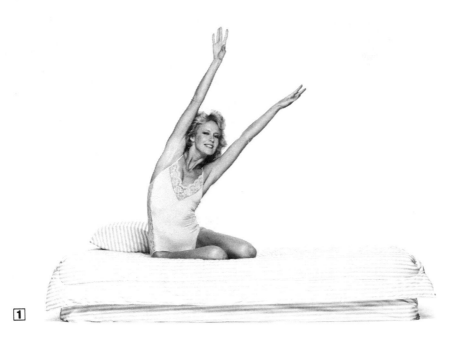

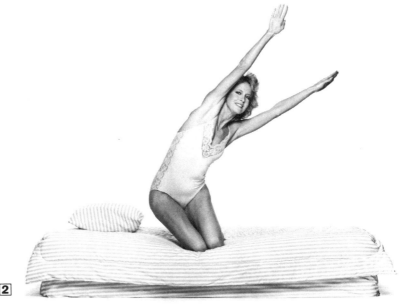

1 Sit erect with your legs tucked behind you to the left, and thrust your arms up high over your head in a left-leaning narrow V.

2 Lift yourself up onto your knees, leaning and stretching your arms up farther to the left.

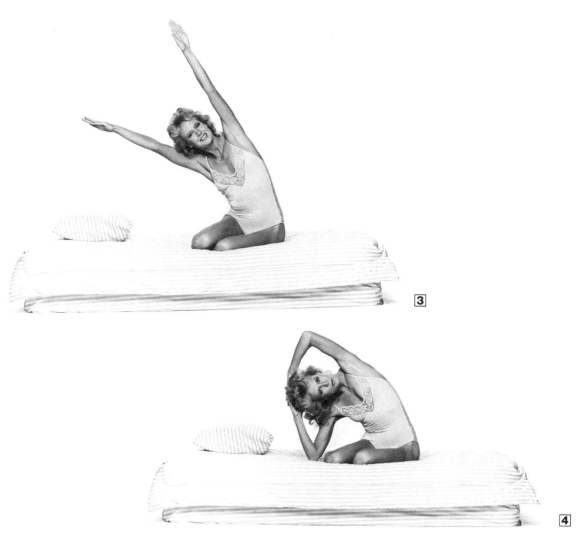

3 Twist your body to the right and sit again, your legs now bent behind you to the right.

4 Clasp your hands on top of your head, and bend your torso down to the right until your right elbow touches the bed.

5 Straighten up to a mirror image of your first position, leaning and stretching now to the right.

6 Repeat the sequence to the opposite side.

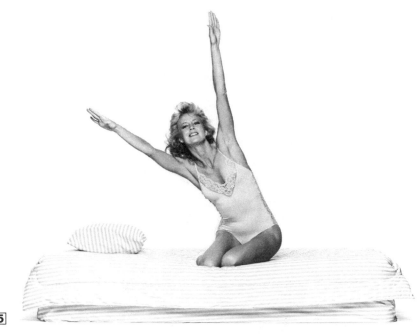

149

Statuesque

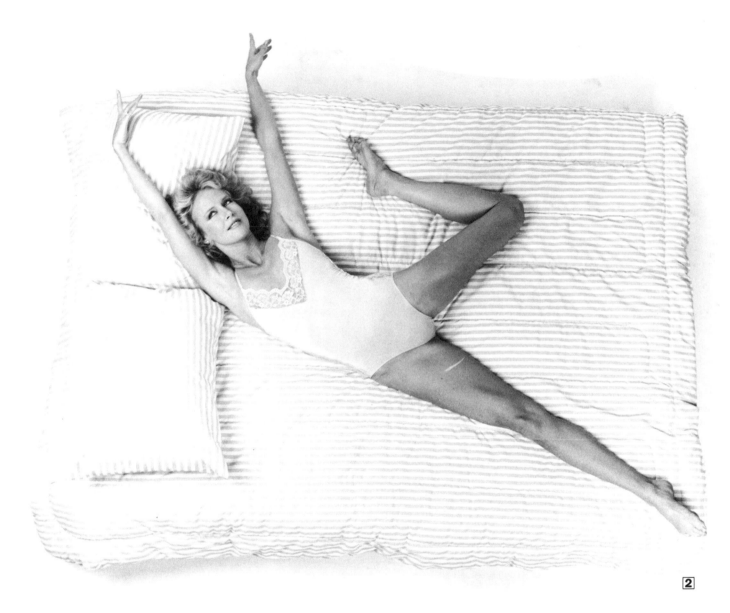

2

1 Lie diagonally across the bed, with your legs together, toes pointed, and your arms stretched slightly to the left over your head, wrists bent to the left, fingers gracefully extended.

2 Bend your left leg up on the bed at a 90-degree angle, so that the sole of your foot faces your head, and hold position for 5 to 10 seconds.

Leg Hold

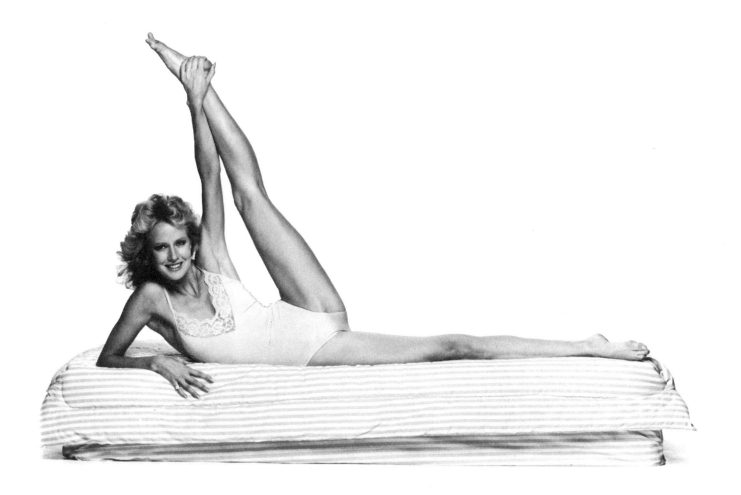

1 Lying on your right side, raise your upper body and support it on your right elbow, slightly above shoulder level, with your forearm flat on the bed, fingers dangling over. Toes pointed, extend your left leg straight up and back toward your head, as high as you can, clasping the heel in your left hand. And again.

2 Repeat the exercise with your right leg.

Splendid Back

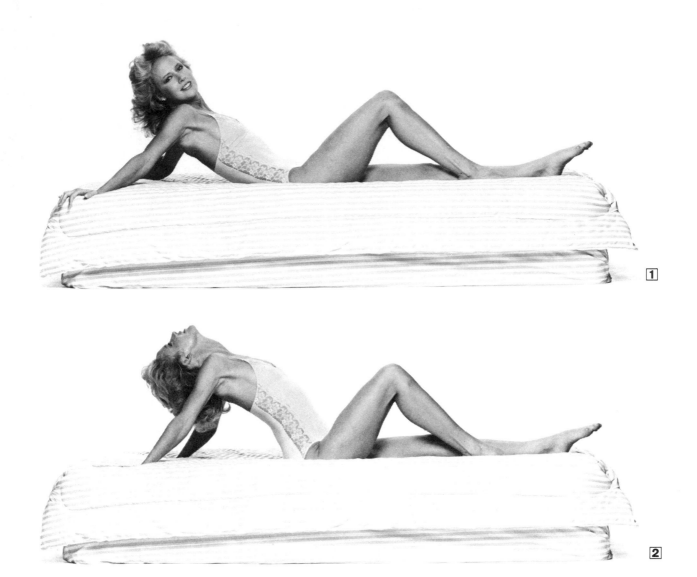

1 Lie back on the end of your spine with your right knee bent up in an inverted V, your torso raised at a slight angle from the bed and supported on your arms spread wide behind you, palms flat on the bed.

2 Arch your back, straightening your elbows and dropping your head back.

Repeat.

Exquisite Split

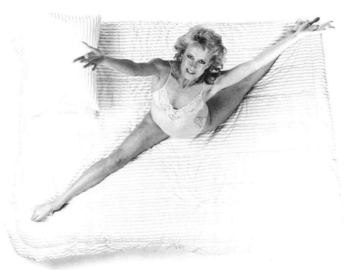

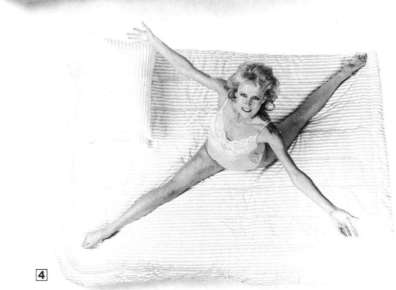

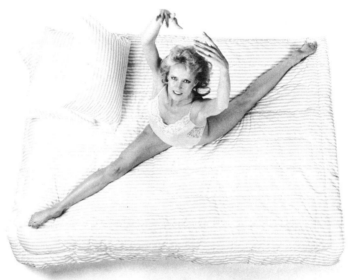

1 In split position diagonally across the bed, sit high, head up, and stretch your arms up and out, palm-up, fingers gracefully extended.

2 Arch your arms gracefully above your head.

3 Extend your arms front and back, parallel to your legs.

4 Spread your arms at shoulder level, straight out to the sides.

5 Reverse the split, and repeat.

Repeat.

In the Kitchen

Nutritional know-how is second nature to my family of athletes. My father grew *living foods* in his garden, and my family thrived on them. Living foods are natural foods, the opposite of packaged, processed, and prepared foods. I call those foods *dead foods* because they don't have the healing and cleansing power of living foods.

When I'm active, my body craves living foods. They taste wonderful and they curb my hunger. They make me feel lively and light, especially when I eat them raw or fast-cooked. When I'm away from home I carry along a plastic bag of fresh fruit or raw vegetables—string beans, carrots, celery, and so on—and they do wonders in keeping my energy level high.

I regard myself as an almost-vegetarian. I rarely eat meat, but I do enjoy fish and dairy products, including yogurt (low-fat, of course). I don't eat refined sugar (it gives you those "sugar blues") but I do use honey sparingly as a sweetener because it has all sorts of minerals and healthful properties. I stay away from salt (who needs high blood pressure and excess water retention?), keep my fat intake low, and I prefer my salads without dressing. (There is nothing like the clean, crisp taste of fresh vegetables.) Add whole grains and whole-grain products to this list, and you have a pretty good idea of what appears on my daily menus and what doesn't.

But face it—I'm human, and there are times when I can't resist the no-no's. When the desire creeps up on me, from time to time I'll succumb and have a ball with an ice cream or a new gourmet recipe. Once-in-a-while can't do any harm, and it keeps my palate interested. Monotony, I think, is the enemy of full enjoyment of life.

Then, to get back on the track I eat my normal healthy foods but cut the amount in half—or lighten up on dinner (*that* meal's the real villain).

I drink a great deal of water. My perception is that most of us don't drink enough. Water is so good for your complexion, eases the whole digestive process, and fills you up so you don't get that craving to overeat. I start the day off with two glasses of water, drink two glasses before each meal, and add at least one more glass before bedtime.

Vitamin supplements play a vital role in my health plan. It's shocking, but true, that by the time a majority of the foods we buy come to our table, most of the vitamins have been depleted. On the number of calories a day that most women consume, the U.S. Department of Agriculture admits you can't get your complete Recommended Daily Allowances (RDAs) of vitamins. Ever since I've been taking multivitamins daily, I've had more energy, needed less sleep, said good-bye to the P.M. lulls; and I've been able to avoid colds and other illnesses.

I don't smoke, I drink rarely, and I cut down on caffeine. I get my highs naturally—from positive thinking, living foods, supportive friends, exercise, and the sports I love.

If you want to know more about my kind of nutrition—the "new nutrition" which is already changing the eating habits and improving the health of millions of people—look into these publications:

Your Personal Vitamin Profile by Dr. Michael Colgan, one of the nation's leading medical nutritionists (William Morrow and Company, New York, 1982). This book is an eye-opening summary of up-to-the-minute developments in all branches of nutrition, not just in the field of vitamins.

All the books by Francine Prince, particularly *Diet for Life* (1980) and *The Best of Francine Prince's Gourmet Diet Recipes* (1982, both published by Simon and Schuster, New York). As far as I'm concerned, Francine Prince wins the gold medal in the Olympics of cooking for better health.

• SUZY GOES BANANAS •

That's not a description of my mental state. It's the name of one of my favorite dishes. Here's the recipe:

> In walnut oil, rapidly sauté chopped pea pods, zucchini, broccoli,
> mushrooms, onions, tomatoes, soybeans, and alfalfa sprouts.
> When almost done, add walnuts and banana slices (*that's* where
> the dish gets its name), and melt in a low-fat pizza cheese.
> Serve on a bed of brown or wild rice. Scrumptious!

And while you're preparing *Suzy Goes Bananas* (or any other dish), why not work out with these exercises?

Plié

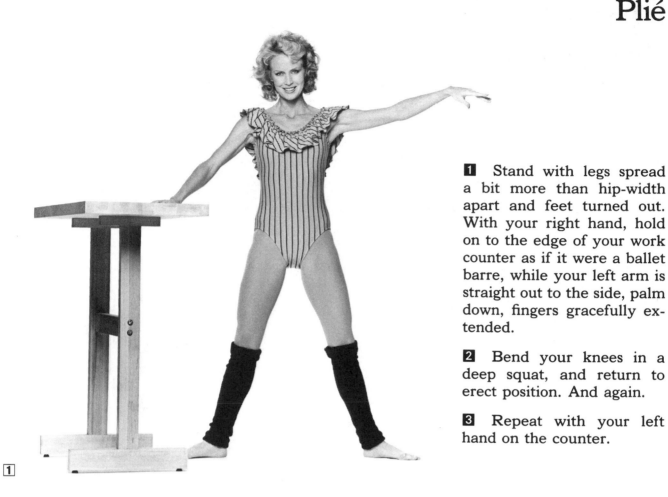

1 Stand with legs spread a bit more than hip-width apart and feet turned out. With your right hand, hold on to the edge of your work counter as if it were a ballet barre, while your left arm is straight out to the side, palm down, fingers gracefully extended.

2 Bend your knees in a deep squat, and return to erect position. And again.

3 Repeat with your left hand on the counter.

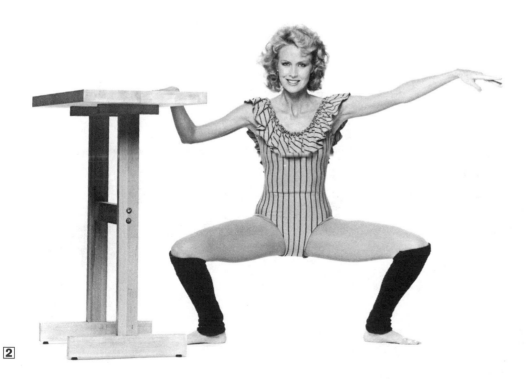

Finger Press Ups

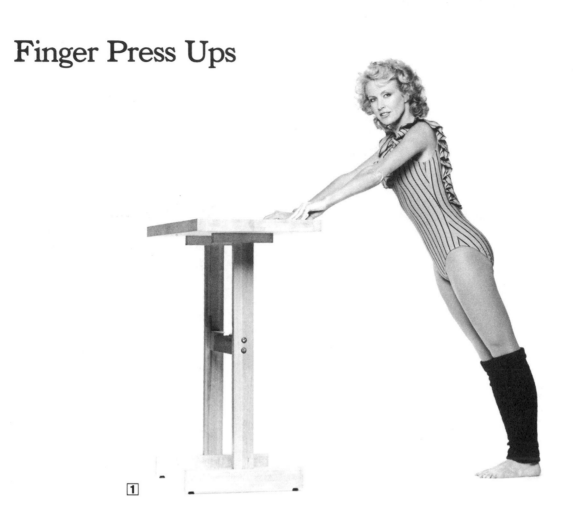

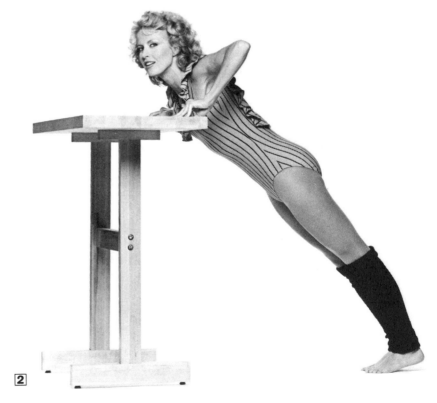

1 Stand a little more than arm's length from work counter and lean toward it, keeping your back and legs straight, your feet together. With your arms straight and wrists up, spread your fingertips on the counter top, your thumbs on the inner edge.

2 Let your heels rise off the floor as you bend your elbows out to the sides and bring your body, still in a straight line, down to the counter edge.

3 Push up to starting position, and repeat.

Back Stretch

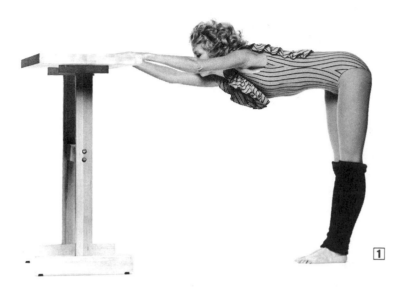

1 With straight legs and feet together, bend forward from the hips so that your back is straight and parallel to the floor, and your hands just reach the work counter, palms flat on the counter top.

2 Bring your head up high as you arch your back down.

3 Arch your back up, head down.

Repeat.

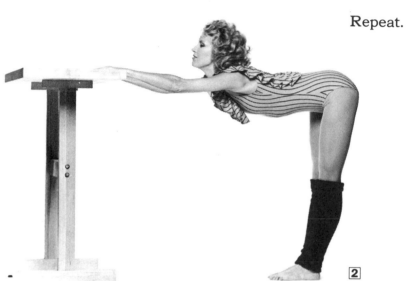

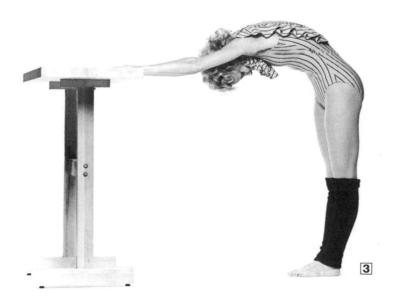

Thigh Lifts

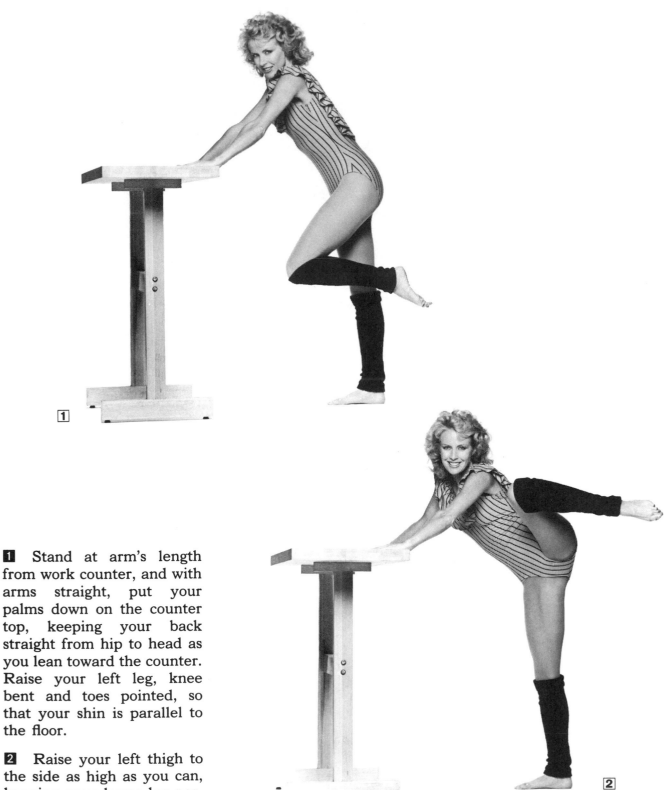

1 Stand at arm's length from work counter, and with arms straight, put your palms down on the counter top, keeping your back straight from hip to head as you lean toward the counter. Raise your left leg, knee bent and toes pointed, so that your shin is parallel to the floor.

2 Raise your left thigh to the side as high as you can, keeping your lower leg parallel to the floor. And again.

3 Repeat exercise with right leg.

Back Bend

1 Stand, with feet slightly apart, at arm's length from work counter, facing away from it, with your fists in the small of your back. Arch your torso backward, looking upside-down at the counter.

2 Reach straight back above your head and grasp the edge of the counter.

3 Tighten your stomach muscles in order to pull yourself back up to starting position.

Repeat.

Note: You may need someone supporting your upper back the first few times you do this exercise.

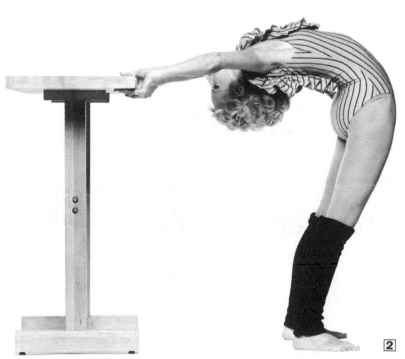

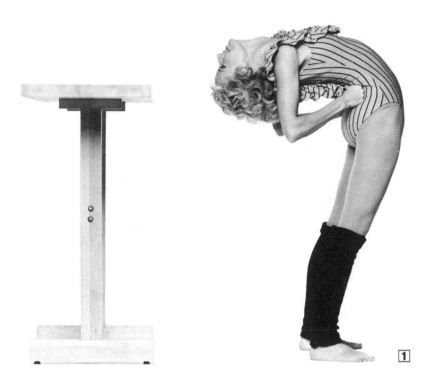

161

Waist Stretch

1 Stand at arm's length from work counter with your left hand grasping the edge, your right arm thrown straight up, palm facing in. Your right leg should be straight, foot turned out. Bring your left foot up, toes pointed, leg straight, and rest your heel on the counter top.

2 Bring your right hand down to grasp your left foot, and your head down to touch your left knee. And again.

3 Repeat, standing on your left leg.

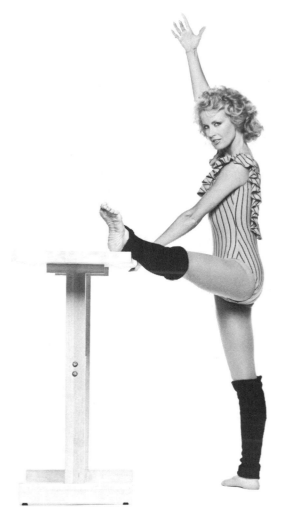

1

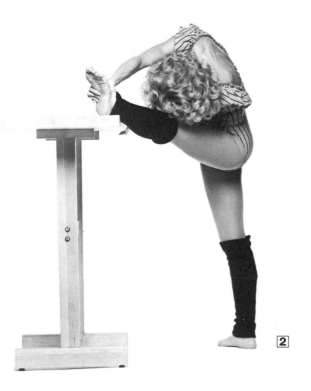

2

Under the Dryer

Looking good and feeling fine—they seem inseparable. That's why I do everything I can to keep myself looking good. I get a good haircut (I cut my hair in layers so it swings), use a light hand with makeup, keep my skin super-clean, baby myself with lots of moisturizer and oils, and use sun screens.

At the end of the day I adore a long languid bath to ease stress and strains on my body and mind. And when things get really rough, I try to have an hour's massage. For me that's the equivalent of getting a day off.

I take especially good care of my hair, because it *is* woman's crowning glory. Because I work out, I need to wash my hair every day, using a conditioner. That could mean dead time under the dryer—but I turn it into live time with, among other things, these exercises.

Downhill Tuck Drying

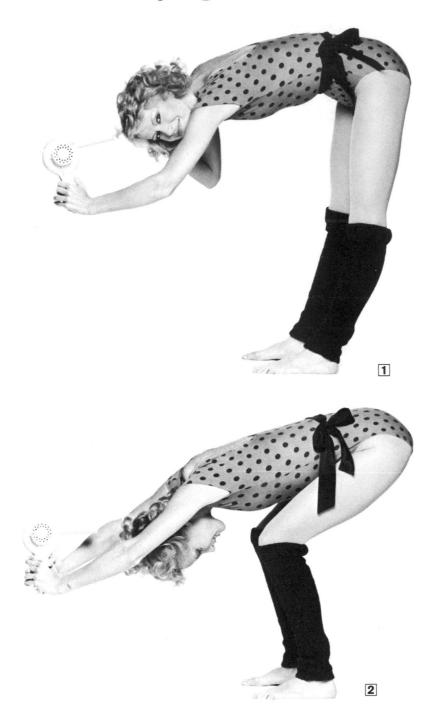

1 With straight legs a few inches apart and feet pointing straight ahead, bend forward from the hips, holding the hand-dryer out in front of you at arm's length—pointing it, of course, at your hair.

2 Bending your knees and keeping your back straight, push your torso down till you're looking back between your legs. Bounce and straighten.

Repeat.

Dry Outrigger

1 Stand erect, legs straight and wide apart, feet turned out, with your hands at the top of your head, the right one holding the hand-dryer.

2 Bend your right knee way out to the side while you dry the right side of your hair.

3 Return to starting position, switch the dryer to your left hand, and repeat the exercise, bending your left knee and drying the left side of your hair. Repeat, alternating, till your hair is all dry.

Improvisation

Provided your hands are free to point the dryer, you can do almost any kind of exercise while you dry your hair. Why not select your favorites, or make up exercises of your own? Creating exercises is as much fun as creating poems or paintings or great recipes.

2

On the Job

I'm a "fitness communicator." That's a designation I originated to describe my mission: to make Americans, particularly American women, realize the importance of sound exercise and good nutrition. I lecture, demonstrate, lobby, write articles, join organizations, host TV shows, do everything I can to bring the gospel of good health to everybody. I even led a march down Pennsylvania Avenue and set up a meeting at the White House to ensure equal opportunity for women in sports in the school system under Title 9. I regard myself as a real "health raiser."

The major reason I've become a fitness communicator is the appalling physical condition of too many Americans. Lower back pain, the major problem among office workers, is almost epidemic. Our jobs have a lot to do with that. "The muscular effort required by most jobs in this country is negligible," says one medical researcher; and unless you're engaged in hard labor, I think you'll agree. Women now represent more than half of the nation's work force, so on-the-job inactivity could be plaguing you too.

But there is a remedy. You can work out while you're at work—and do it unobtrusively—with these exercises I've designed for you. It's a fun way to recharge your battery when you need it most, and give you a sense of humor.

Scissors

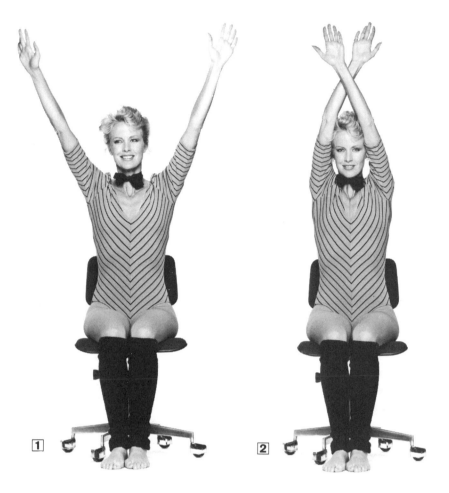

1 Sitting in a chair with your legs and feet close together, raise your arms in a wide V over your head, palms forward, fingers spread.

2 Crisscross your arms in a scissorlike motion while you bring them gradually down to shoulder level, stretched out in front of you.

3 Extend your arms out to the sides, palms down.

4 Keeping your arms straight, continue to crisscross them as you bring them down in front of you to your knees, and up again.

Repeat.

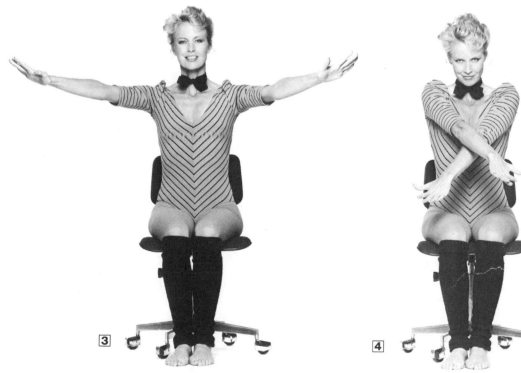

Collapse

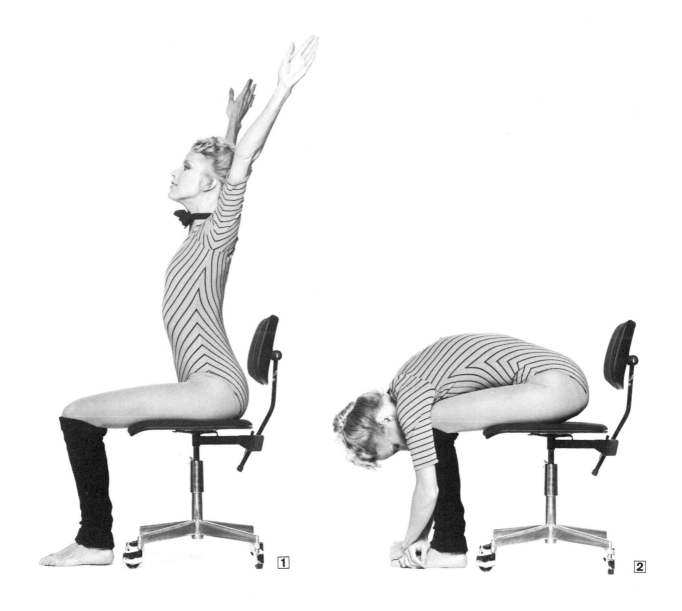

1 Sit high in your chair with your legs and feet close together, and fling your arms up and out in a wide V above your head. Inhale deeply.

2 Collapse forward till your head hangs over your knees and your hands are loosely crossed on your feet. Exhale and relax.

Repeat.

Jazz Shoulders

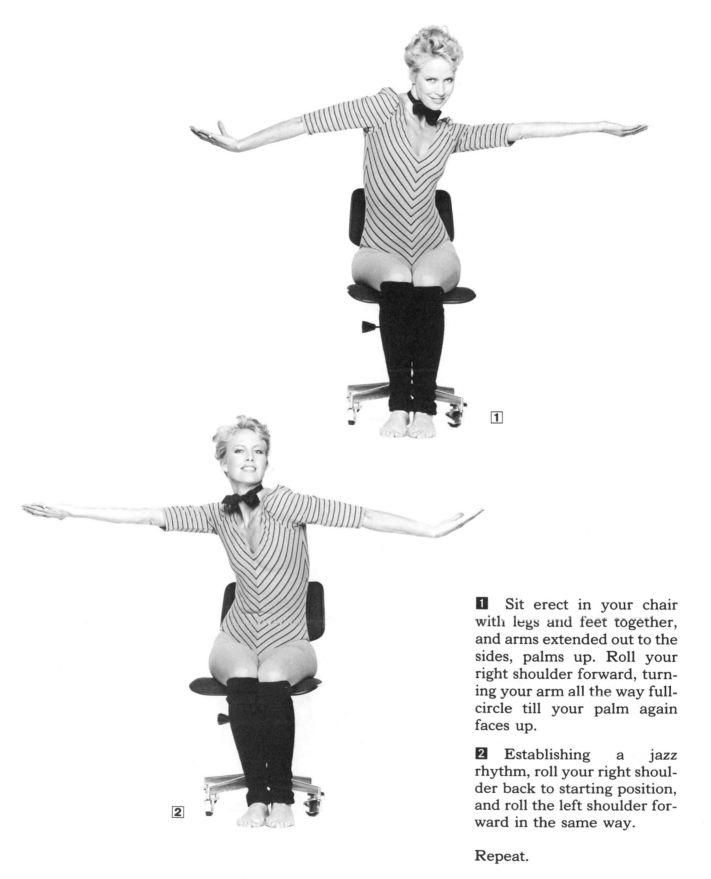

1 Sit erect in your chair with legs and feet together, and arms extended out to the sides, palms up. Roll your right shoulder forward, turning your arm all the way full-circle till your palm again faces up.

2 Establishing a jazz rhythm, roll your right shoulder back to starting position, and roll the left shoulder forward in the same way.

Repeat.

169

Waist Stretch

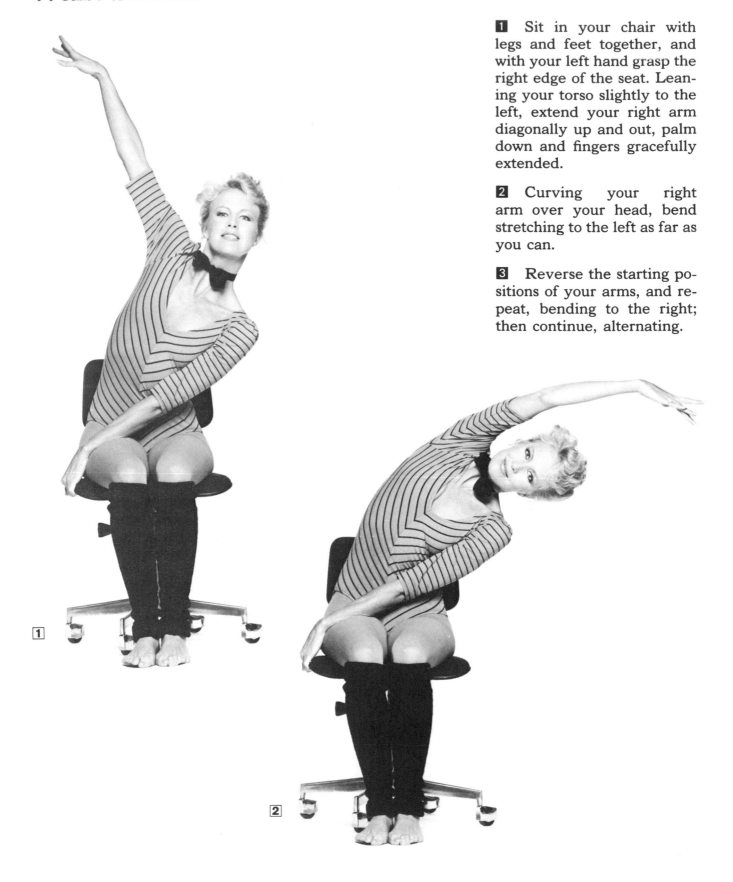

1 Sit in your chair with legs and feet together, and with your left hand grasp the right edge of the seat. Leaning your torso slightly to the left, extend your right arm diagonally up and out, palm down and fingers gracefully extended.

2 Curving your right arm over your head, bend stretching to the left as far as you can.

3 Reverse the starting positions of your arms, and repeat, bending to the right; then continue, alternating.

Back Stretch

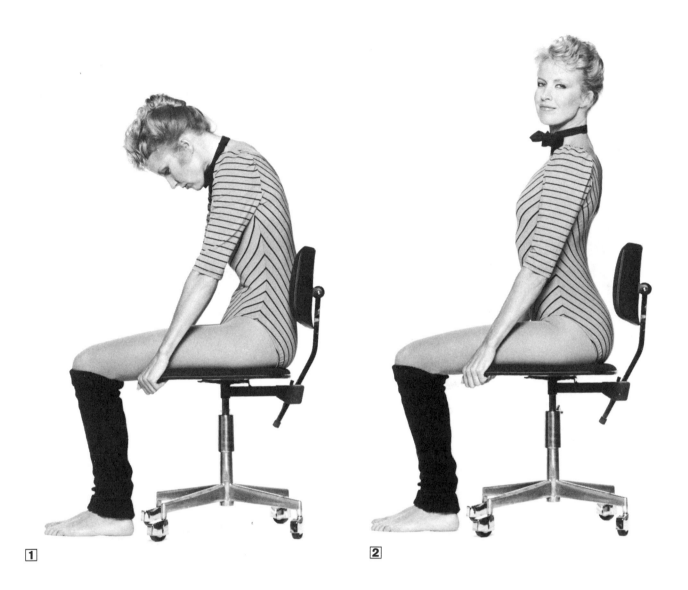

1   Sit in your chair with legs and feet together, back straight, and grasp the front edge of the seat with both hands. Let your head and shoulders slump forward.

2   Without letting go of the seat, arch your back and sit up tall, head high.

Repeat.

Chair Abdominal

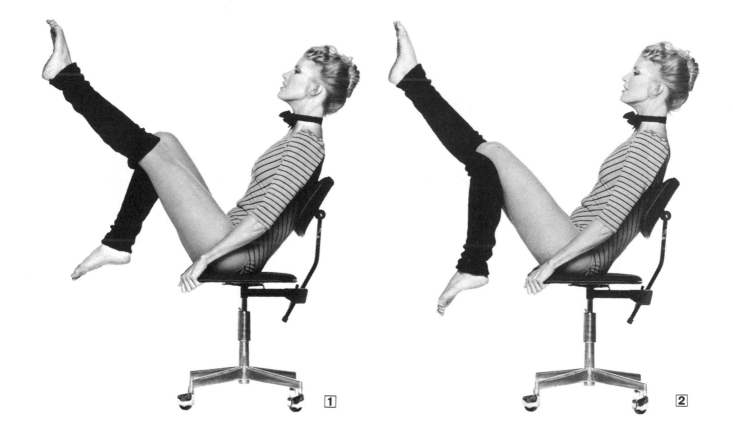

1 Sit on the edge of the chair, leaning diagonally back against the chair back and grasping the front edge of the seat with both hands. Raise your legs to form a V with your torso, right leg bent at the knee, left leg up and straight, toes pointed.

2 Straighten your right leg and bend your left, reversing your original position; then alternate.

Back Twist

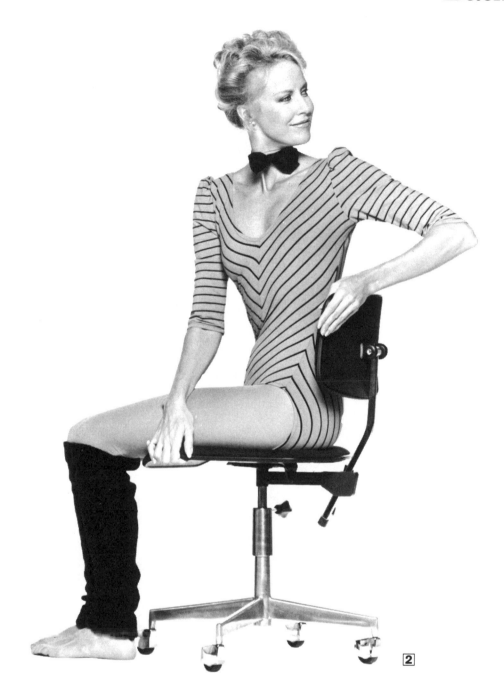

2

1 Sit in a chair with your knees and feet together. With your right arm, grasp the left front edge of the seat, while your left hand grips the left top back of the chair.

2 Twisting your upper body to the left, look back over your left shoulder.

3 Reverse the position of your arms, and twist to your right.

Repeat.

While Waiting

Do you realize how much waiting time there is in all our lives—waiting for a bus, waiting in check-out lines, waiting for the toast to pop—waiting, waiting, waiting. I hate waiting, don't you? So, don't wait any longer; turn waiting time into active time with these exercises.

I Don't Know

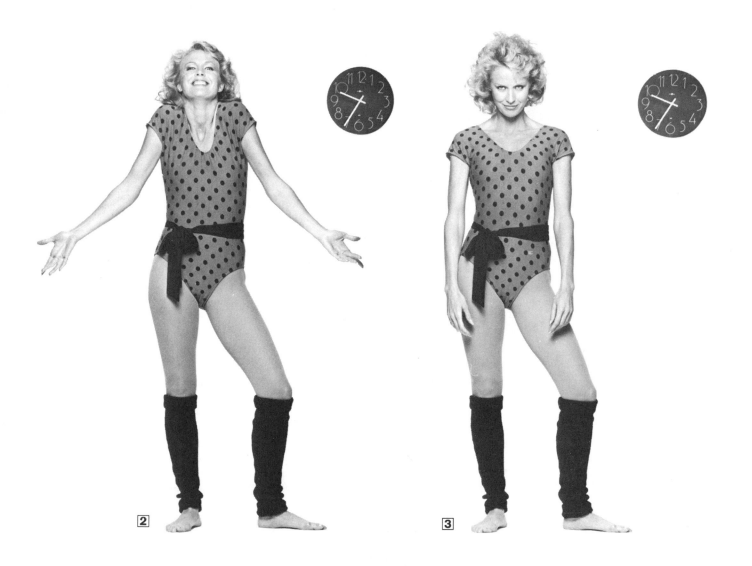

1 Stand relaxed, with right leg straight, left leg and foot turned out, knee bent, arms at sides.

2 Lift your shoulders in a tight shrug, spreading your arms out from your sides, palms up.

3 Lower head. Drop your shoulders, relax your neck, and let your arms hang loosely.

Repeat.

Toe-Ups

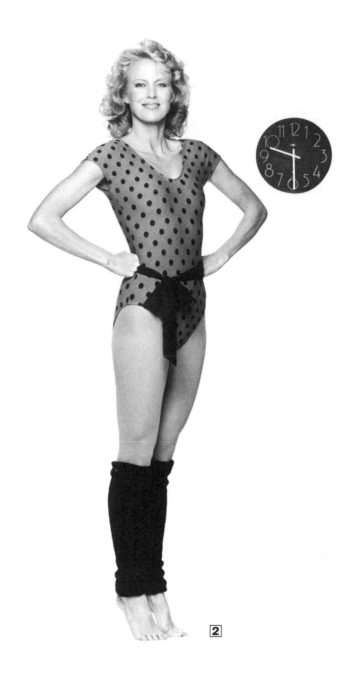

2

1 Stand erect, arms akimbo with fists at your waist, and legs together.

2 Rise high on your toes, and repeat.

Lug Your Luggage

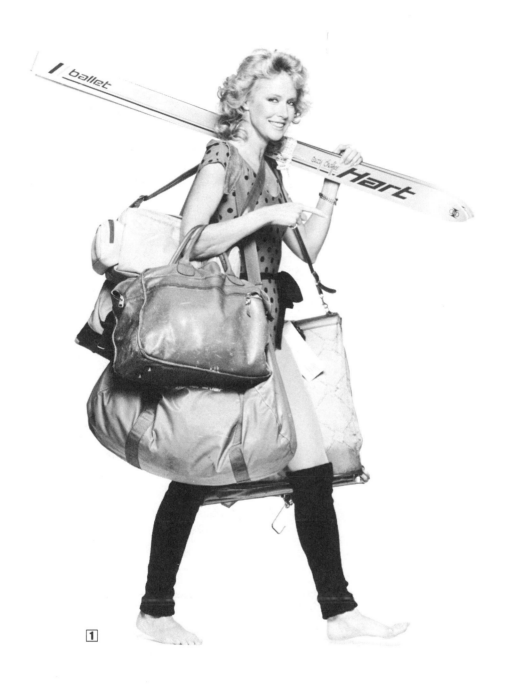

1 Just walking around, carrying heavy luggage, is pretty good exercise.

Stretching for the News

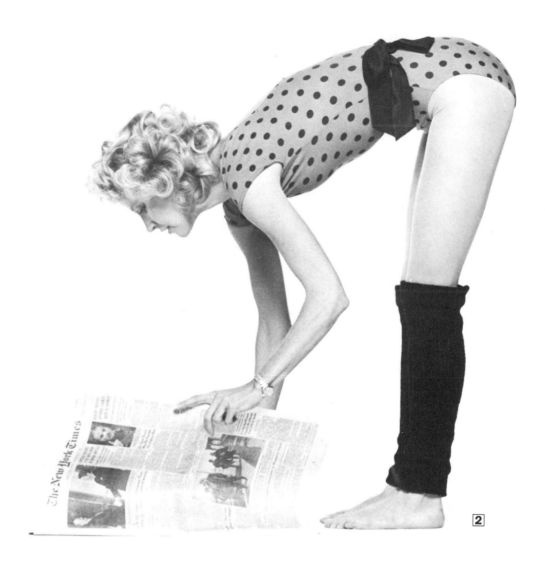

1 Drop a newspaper on the floor in front of you, and stand erect, legs and feet together, arms at your sides.

2 Bending forward from the hips and keeping your legs straight, flip through the newspaper.

Sitting on the Wall

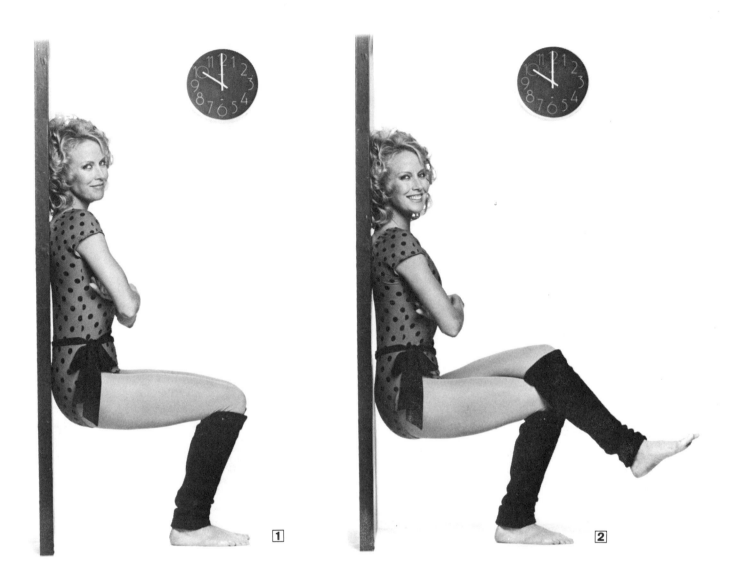

1 With your back flat against a wall from head to hip, and your arms folded across your chest, sit on the air as if it were a straight chair, with your legs together, thighs parallel to the floor, and your feet turned slightly out.

2 Cross your left leg over the right, alternately pointing and flexing your toes.

3 Now cross your right leg over the left; then alternate.

Calf Stretch

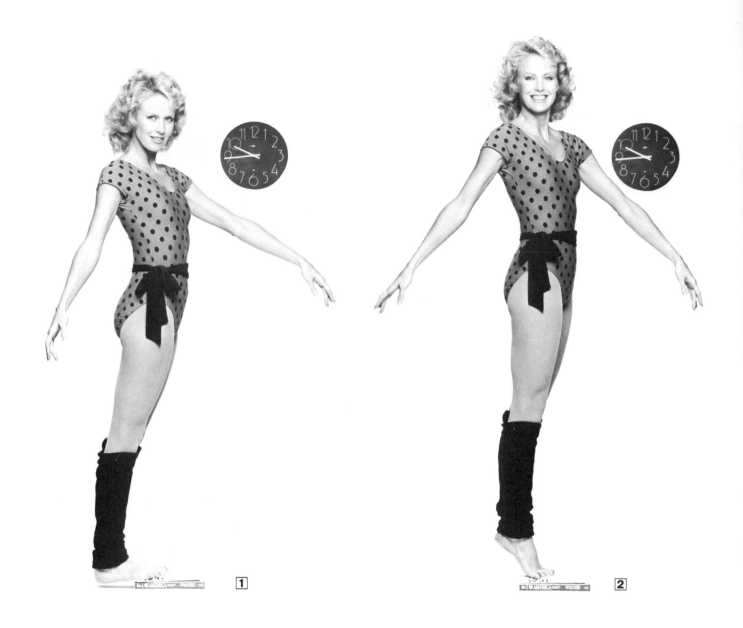

1 Stack a couple of books on the floor and stand erect on them on the balls of your feet, so that your heels are off the floor. Your arms should be spread wide for balance, your legs and feet together.

2 Now up on your toes, and repeat.

Pirouette

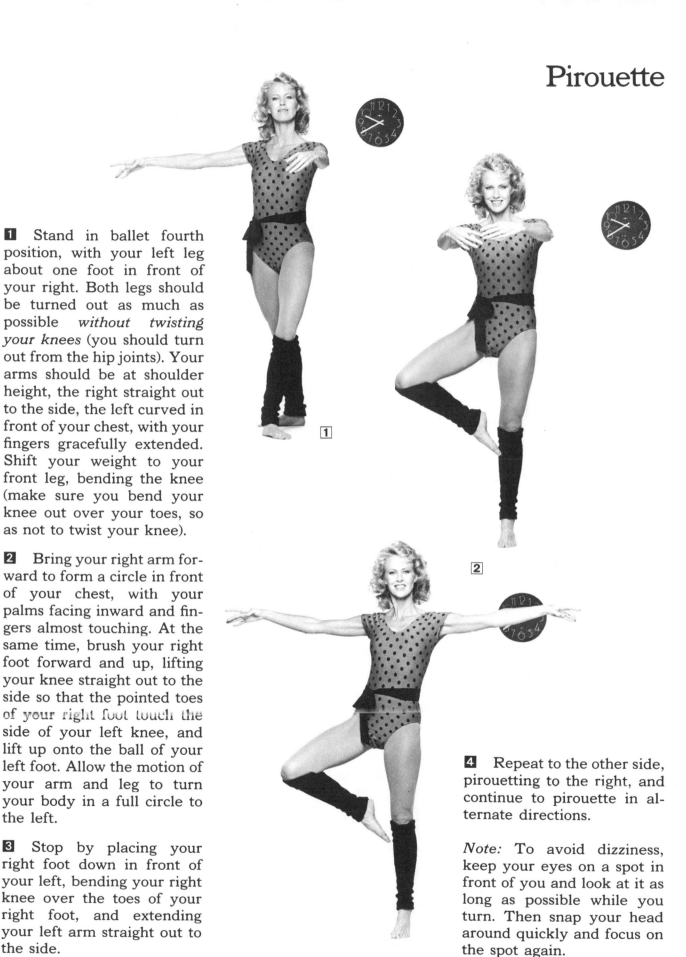

1 Stand in ballet fourth position, with your left leg about one foot in front of your right. Both legs should be turned out as much as possible *without twisting your knees* (you should turn out from the hip joints). Your arms should be at shoulder height, the right straight out to the side, the left curved in front of your chest, with your fingers gracefully extended. Shift your weight to your front leg, bending the knee (make sure you bend your knee out over your toes, so as not to twist your knee).

2 Bring your right arm forward to form a circle in front of your chest, with your palms facing inward and fingers almost touching. At the same time, brush your right foot forward and up, lifting your knee straight out to the side so that the pointed toes of your right foot touch the side of your left knee, and lift up onto the ball of your left foot. Allow the motion of your arm and leg to turn your body in a full circle to the left.

3 Stop by placing your right foot down in front of your left, bending your right knee over the toes of your right foot, and extending your left arm straight out to the side.

4 Repeat to the other side, pirouetting to the right, and continue to pirouette in alternate directions.

Note: To avoid dizziness, keep your eyes on a spot in front of you and look at it as long as possible while you turn. Then snap your head around quickly and focus on the spot again.

Close to Nature

When I want to clear my head I climb a mountain, and when I get to the top I exercise and meditate. I feel wonderment, appreciation, peace, and love. I feel a power, a spirit. Then my problems melt away. I can enjoy this elevating experience as well on a secluded beach, taking a walk in the country, anywhere close to nature. Perhaps you can too.

But if this kind of spiritual adventure is not for you, you can still get a special thrill exercising in the great outdoors. I've designed two sets of close-to-nature workouts—one for the beach, the other for among trees and growing things—which will help you bloom as freely as any of nature's beauties.

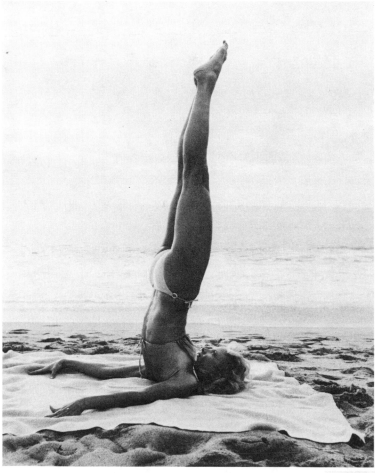

 1

Shoulder Stand

1 Lying on your back, with your arms flat at your sides, palms down, raise your torso and legs straight up in the air, toes pointed, so that your weight rests on your shoulders.

2 Bend your right knee down toward your head; then straighten your leg up again.

3 Bend your left knee down toward your head and up again; then continue, alternating legs.

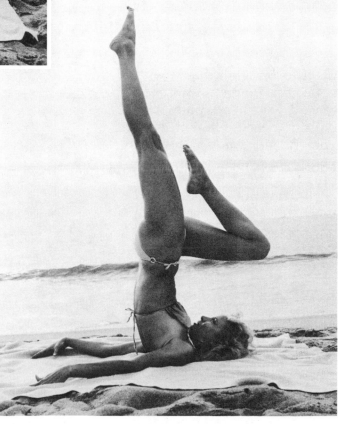

2

183

Bridge to Back-Bend Up

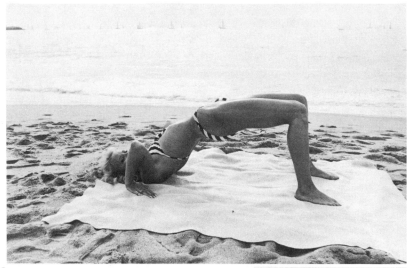

1

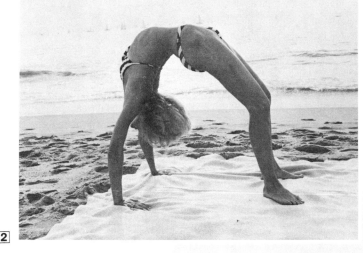

2

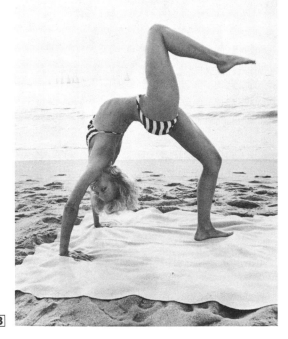

3

1 Lie on your back with your arms bent out and back toward your head, palms flat on the beach blanket with your fingers pointing toward your feet. Raise your body off the ground till it is supported on your shoulders and your turned-out feet, with your lower legs, about hip-width apart, at right angles to the ground.

2 Straighten your arms, raising your upper torso till your whole body forms an arch.

3 Holding the back arch, lift your right leg up, knee bent, toes pointed.

184

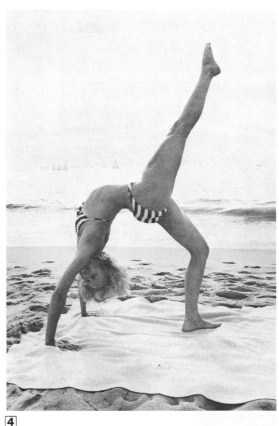

4 Carry the upward motion through, straightening your leg, and pointing your toes up toward the sky; then return your right foot to the ground.

5 Pushing up with your hands, pull your torso up, using your stomach muscles and the momentum of your hips. Keep looking back until you come up to a standing position. Finish high on your toes, arms spread wide above your head.

Repeat.

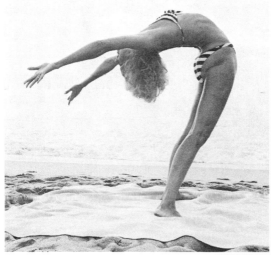

Split Warmup

This is the prelude to one of my favorite beach exercises, the Slide in Sand Split, which follows.

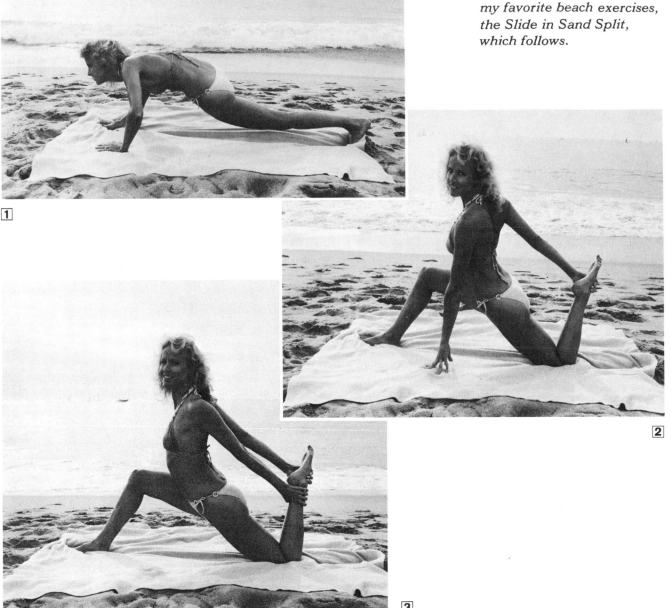

1 On a beach blanket, go into a low "on your marks" crouch, supporting yourself on flat palms, with your right foot between your hands, and your left leg extended way back, knee off the ground.

2 Lower your left knee to the blanket and, supporting yourself on the fingertips of your straight left arm, raise your torso to an erect position. Reach your right hand back to grasp your left foot, lifting the lower leg in a V formation.

3 Reach back your left hand as well, and grasp your left ankle.

4 Reverse your starting position and repeat, grasping your right foot.

Slide in Sand Split

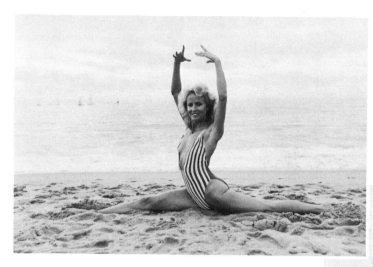

1

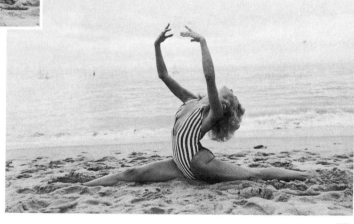

2

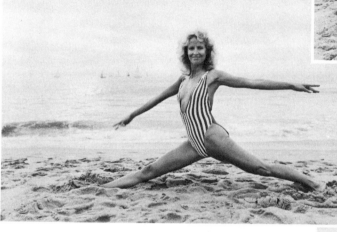

3

1 Arms extended to the sides, slide into a split position in the sand, lowering your hands to the ground.

2 In split position, stretch up high and arch your arms over your head, fingers gracefully extended.

3 Lean your head way back, arching your back like a bow.

Repeat.

Cartwheel

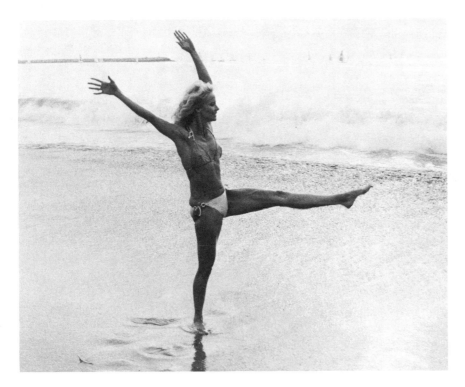

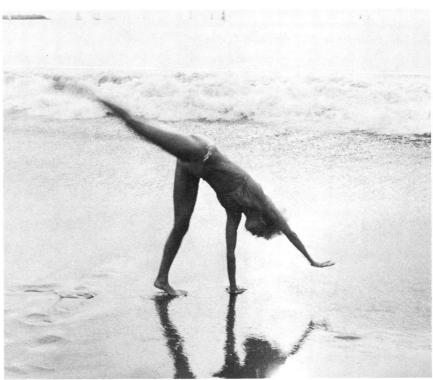

1 Turning cartwheels at the edge of the water is more fun than anything.

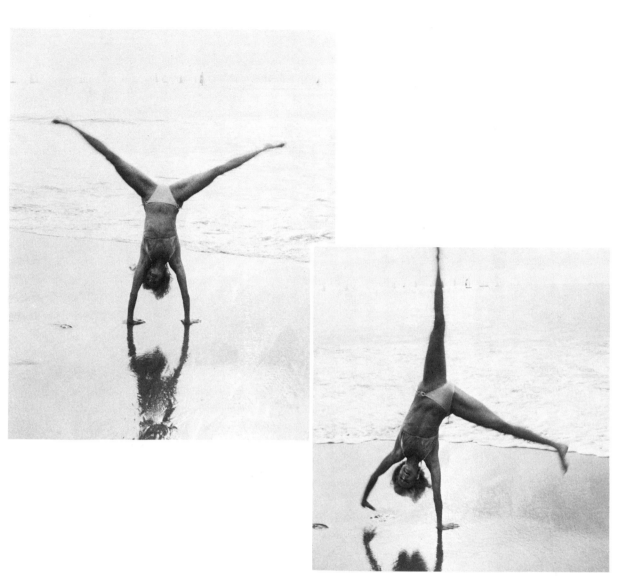

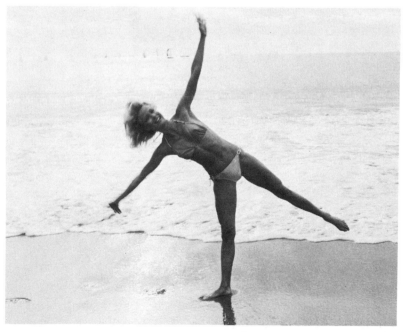

Super Loop and Roll

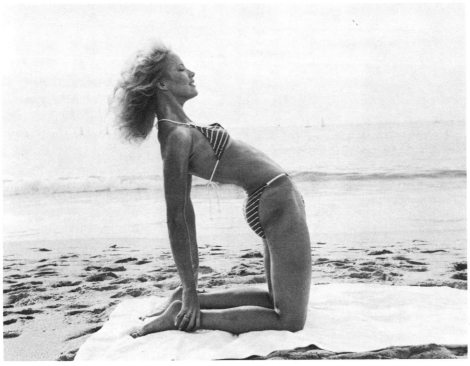

1 Kneeling up with head erect, legs slightly apart, lean your torso back from the hips and grasp your ankles behind you.

2 Bring your head way back, as far as you can, arching your back in and forming a sort of rectangular loop.

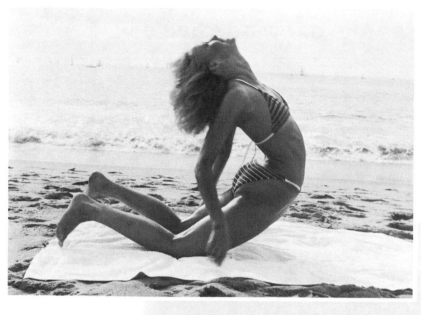

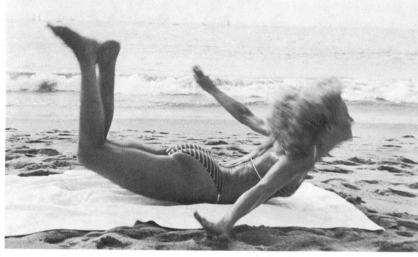

3 Release your hold on your ankles, and roll your body forward, knees to hips to stomach, in rocking-horse fashion, finishing with your head erect, your arms flung up and out behind you, your legs reaching up from the hips as high as they will go.

Repeat.

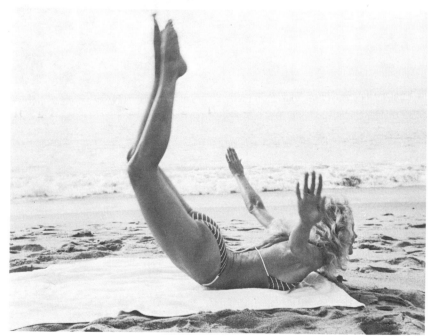

Calf Stretch

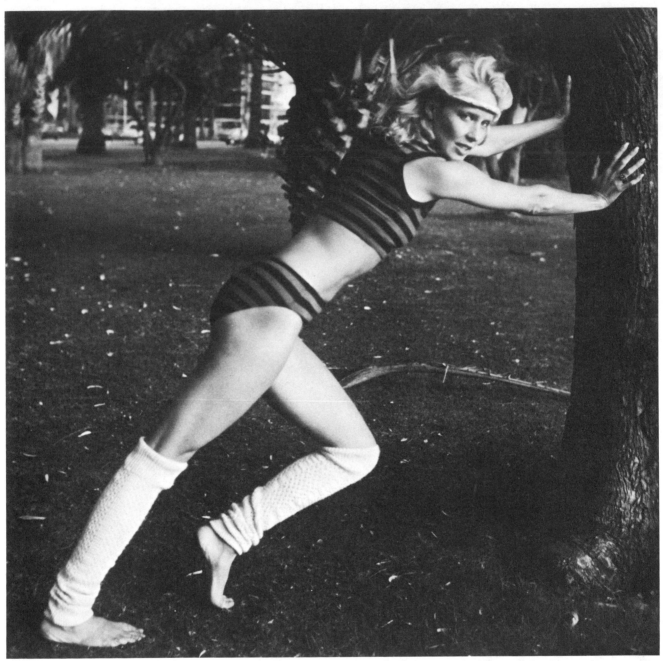

2

1 Find yourself a big tree and lean your palms against it, at arm's length, moving your feet back till you are leaning against the tree at a straight diagonal.

2 Walk in place, raising first one heel, then the other from the ground, pushing against the tree trunk with your hands and stretching the calf muscles of the back leg.

Waist Stretch

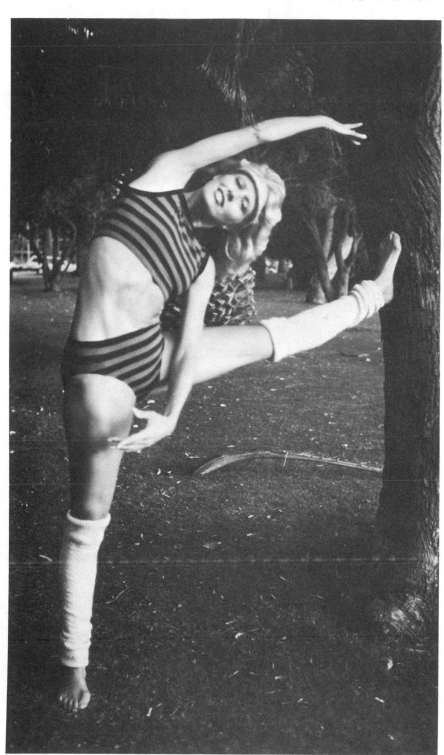

1 Standing on your right leg, foot turned out, raise your left leg straight out at right angles toward the tree, pressing the sole of your foot against the tree, toes up. With your right arm arched above your head, and your left curved forward across your body, fingers gracefully extended, bend stretching toward the tree as far down as you can. And again.

2 Face the other way, raise your right leg, and repeat.

Standing Leg Hold

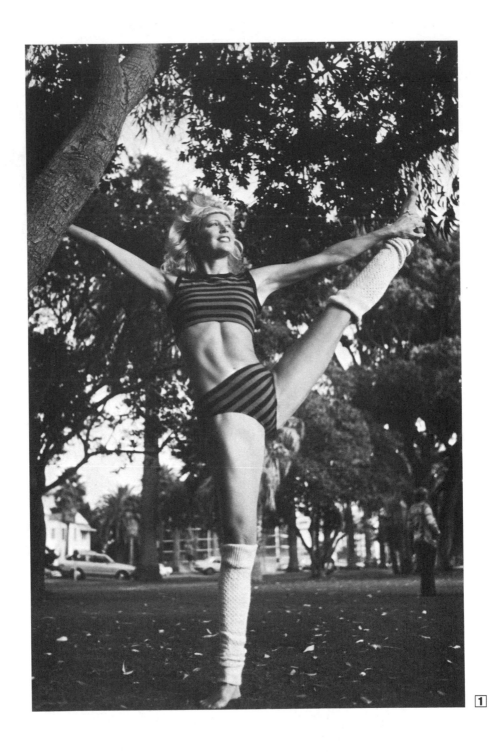

1 Find a sturdy branch to hold on to at about head height, grasp it with your right hand, and stand straight on your right leg, foot turned slightly out. Raise your left leg diagonally up, toes pointed, and clasp the ankle, at arm's length, in your left hand.

2 Repeat with your right leg; then continue, alternating legs.

Park Bench Abdominal

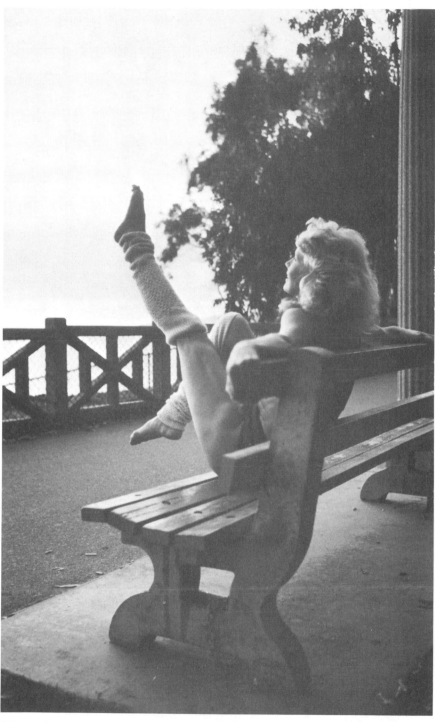

1

1 Sit on the edge of a bench, leaning back diagonally against the back of the bench, with your arms stretched out along the back, your hands holding on to the top of the bench back. Raise your legs to form a V with your torso, right leg bent at the knee, left leg up and straight, toes pointed.

2 Straighten your right leg and bend your left, reversing your original position; then alternate.

VI

Exercises with the Man in Your Life

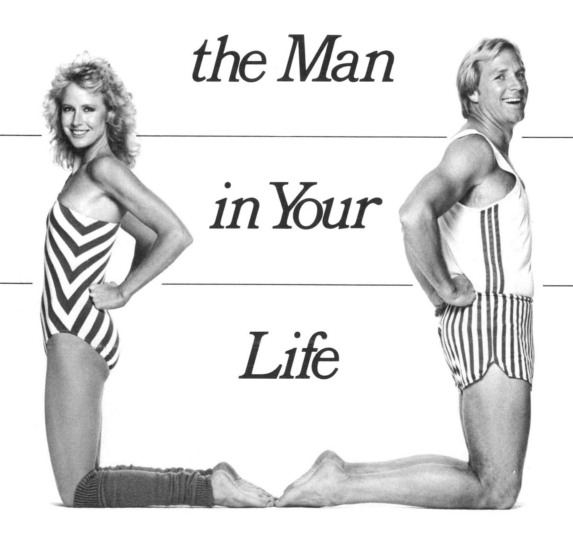

$\mathbf{F}$itness can be such a great goal for a couple, something to reach for and find together. It's a joint venture in sharing the joys of health and good looks. It's an expression of love, and a wonderful form of sex play. And, if he's not already fit, it's a way of avoiding the resentment of the man in your life as he sees you build a trim youthful body and an active, exuberant personality while he remains in a sedentary rut, piling on age, weight, and lethargy.

The man in these pictures is Tom Lewis. You can catch him on the slopes of Aspen when he's not running his Florida-based conglomerate. He wanted no part of exercises that bore him, so I invented these very special fun ones. They will build strength (especially for you) and flexibility (especially for your partner)— and you'll have a ball doing them. Exercising with a partner can be twice as much fun.

There's no need for detailed descriptions of these exercises. What you see is what you'll do.

The Waisted Arch

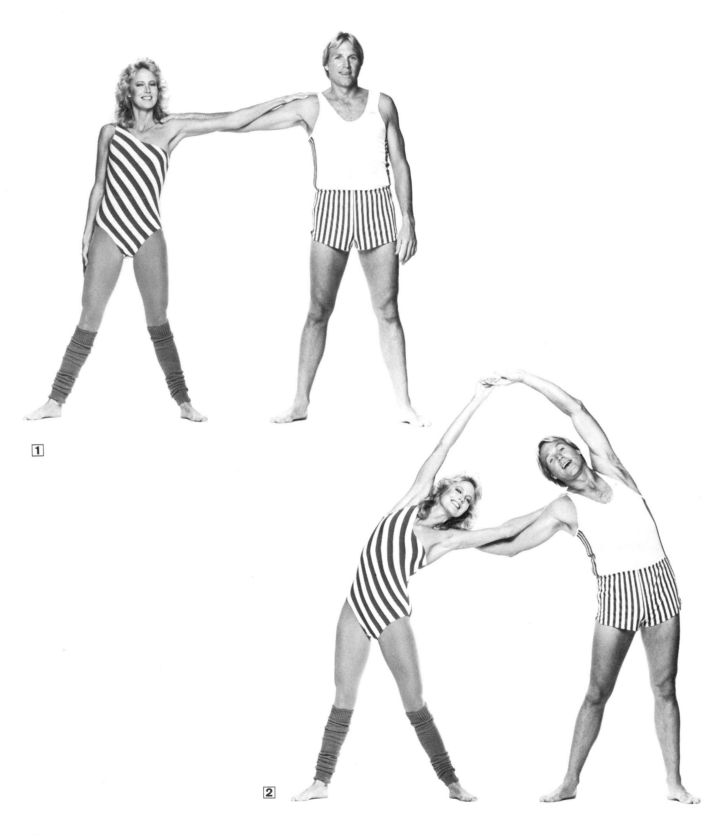

1

2

Reach for higher things together, and your waistline will shape up.

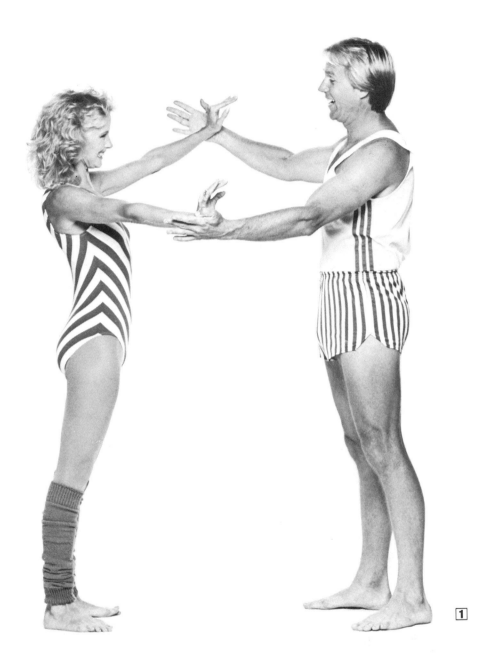

Being in each other's arms can be as healthful as it's joyful—even when one of you puts up a show of resistance.

Split Resistance

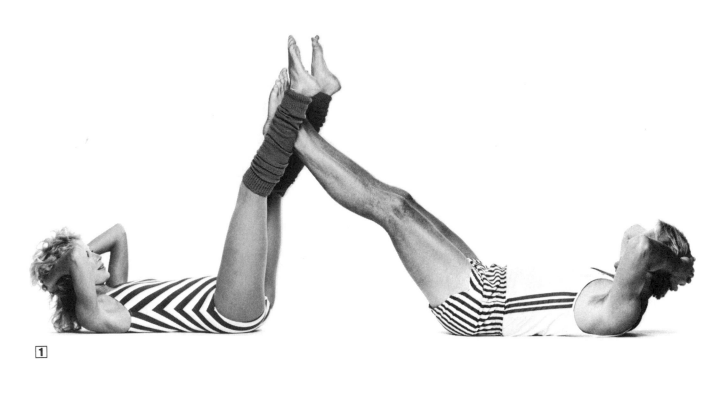

1

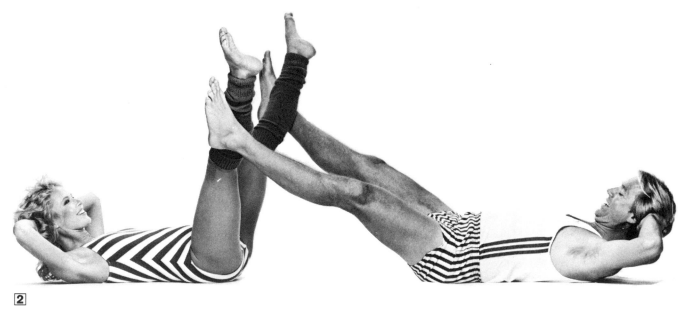

2

First you use your legs to resist his efforts to split, and then it's vice-versa.

Heavy Toe-Ups

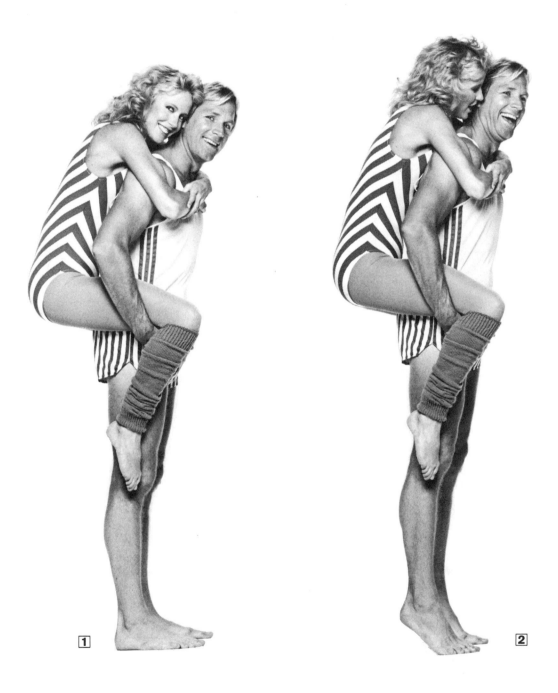

I've heard it said that a man has to have a woman on his back to get him on his toes. And here it works the other way around, too. Try it.

Two on a Seesaw

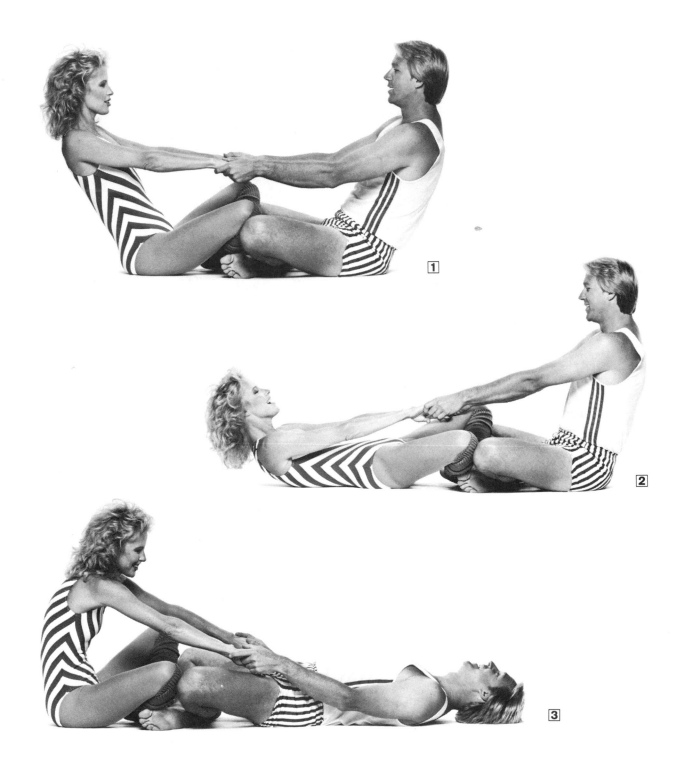

1

2

3

Every relationship between the sexes has its ups and downs. But here, even when you're down it's good for you.

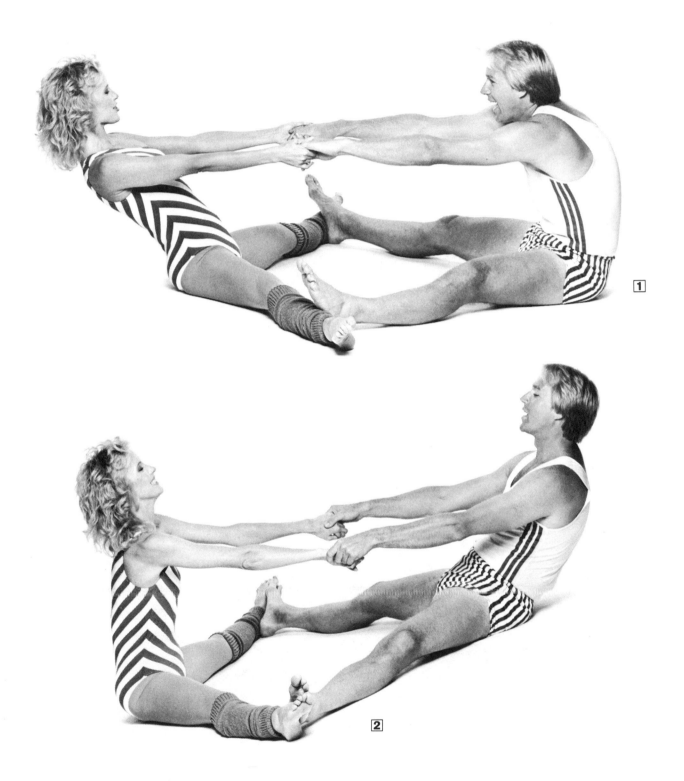

This split stretch is a tug-o'-war between the sexes. Sometimes you win and sometimes he wins, but when the exercise is over, both of you win.

Linked Sit-Ups

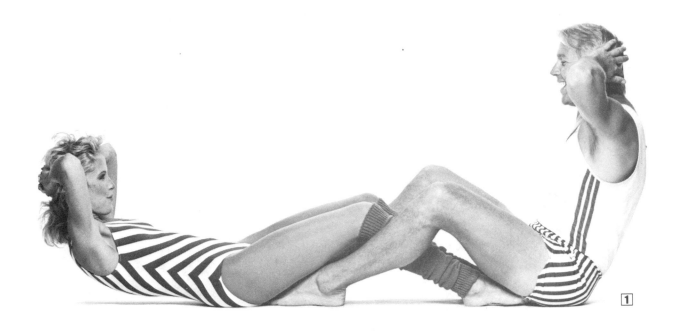

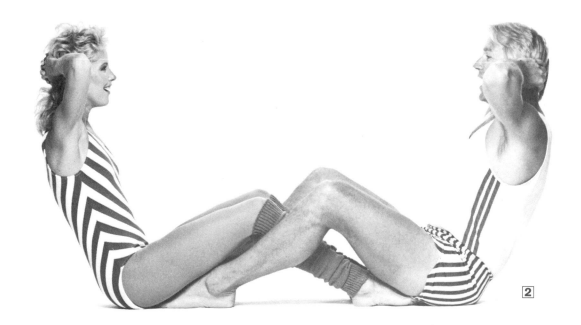

Each partner supplies the leverage for the other to get up in the world. Which is the way it should be, isn't it?

Arc de Triomphe

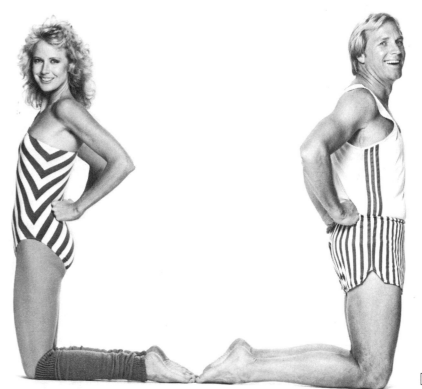

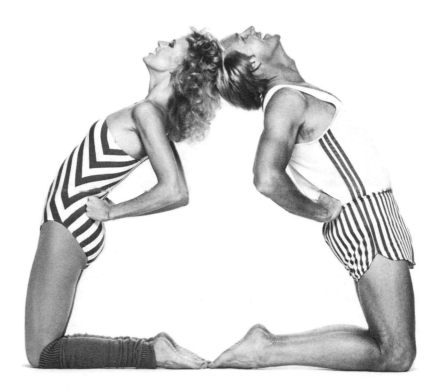

Or—a triumphant meeting of minds.

Side-Ups

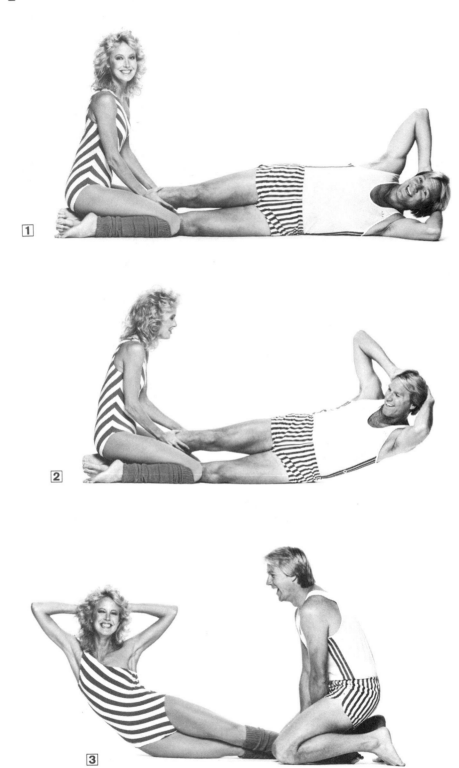

What you're doing here is sitting on his legs to give him leverage when he does his side-ups. He'll do the same for you.

Back Stretch

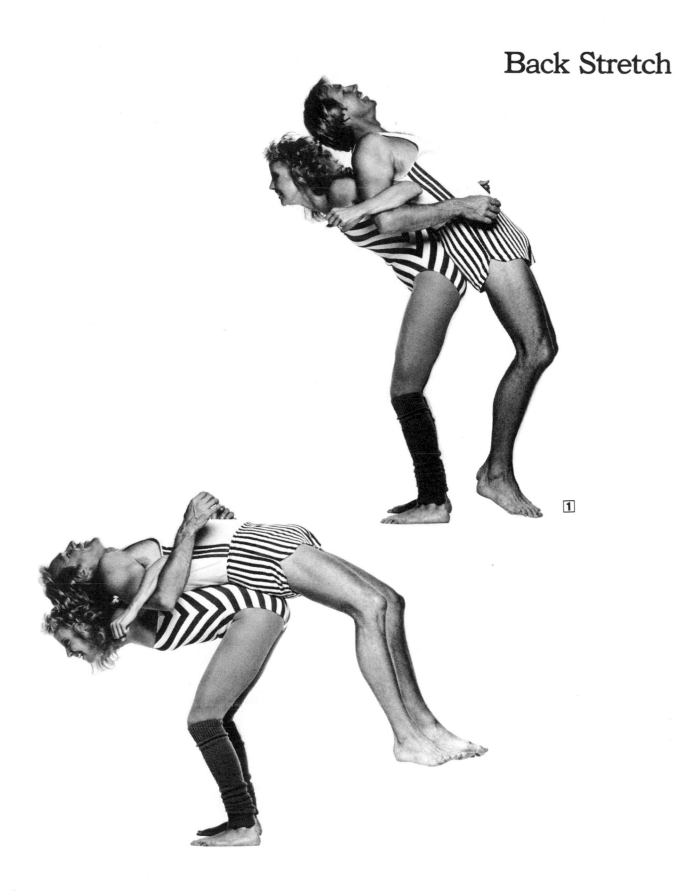

Who says a woman can't carry her own weight in this world? And a man's weight too? Now see if he can carry yours.

VII

Exercises

for

Super-Moms

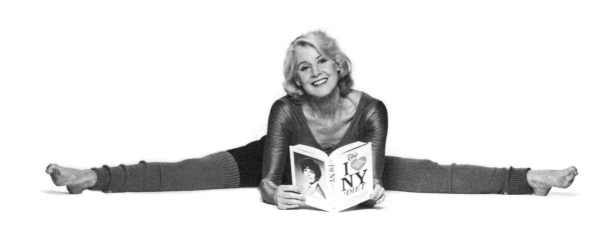

My mother was on the Olympic ski squad but drifted away from athletics in later life. She developed severe progressive asthma, was hospitalized frequently, and often had to depend on a special breathing machine. Breathing became such an ordeal that she resigned herself to dying.

She had seen numerous doctors. All prescribed medication, but only two suggested additional natural therapy like walking and drinking water. Not one doctor asked what she ate, or made any attempt to link her possible recovery with good nutrition. One hospital doctor even denied her permission to consult with the staff physical therapist, and took away her natural vitamins, because "the food here is so good." It was just the opposite. She was served white bread, white rice, canned and processed foods with preservatives, and not one fresh fruit or vegetable. The sweet desserts gave her such a sugar high that it took her weeks to get off the sugar blues. She put on weight, lost energy.

My mother had done so much for me in my life that I decided to reverse roles. With much love, I persuaded her to get into a regular fitness program. She enjoyed it, and took on a new responsibility: getting healthy and staying healthy. She studied preventive medicine, and learned that with the right nutrition and the right exercises, she could help control asthma. And she did it. Other older people have won their battles against disease the same way.

Within a year of her new fitness program, my Super-Mom—aged sixty-four then—learned to do a beautiful split, and performed a double gymnastic routine with me in a President's Council on Physical Fitness film and in a TV spot I wrote promoting the Olympics. Recently she participated in the ten-kilometer walk-and-jog race in Bermuda, and the ten-kilometer cross-country ski race at Sugarbush, Vermont. Ten kilometers is a bit more than six miles. And she won!

Then, after fifteen years away from skis, she put on (for safety) a shorter pair of the lighter-weight skis I designed for women, and raced with me in the Suzy Chaffee Celebrity Pro-Am, making a sensational comeback. Mom's attitude used to be "When I get older, why try?" Now it's "Why quit?"

Now meet my Super-Mom at seventy, as she demonstrates the exercises that can help make any older woman look and feel young again.

Weighty Books

My Super-Mom believes there's no sense spending money on weights when you have a couple of good hardcovers in the house. Here she builds strength and helps keep slim with, appropriately, two excellent diet books.

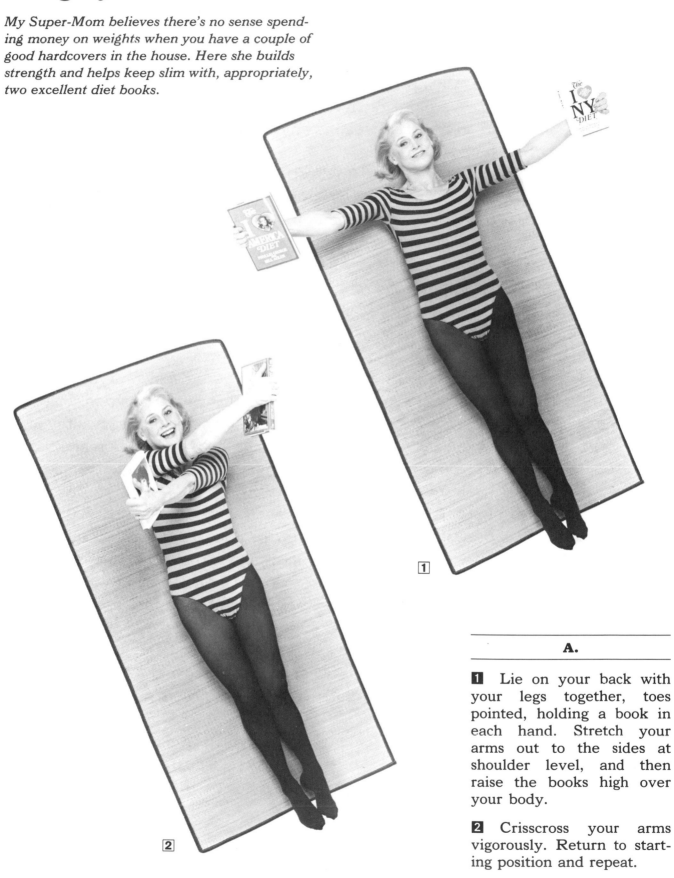

1

2

A.

1 Lie on your back with your legs together, toes pointed, holding a book in each hand. Stretch your arms out to the sides at shoulder level, and then raise the books high over your body.

2 Crisscross your arms vigorously. Return to starting position and repeat.

B.

1 Extend your arms diagonally, left arm up, right arm down. Then bring the books together high above your body at shoulder level.

2 Repeat, starting with your right arm up, the left down; then continue, alternating.

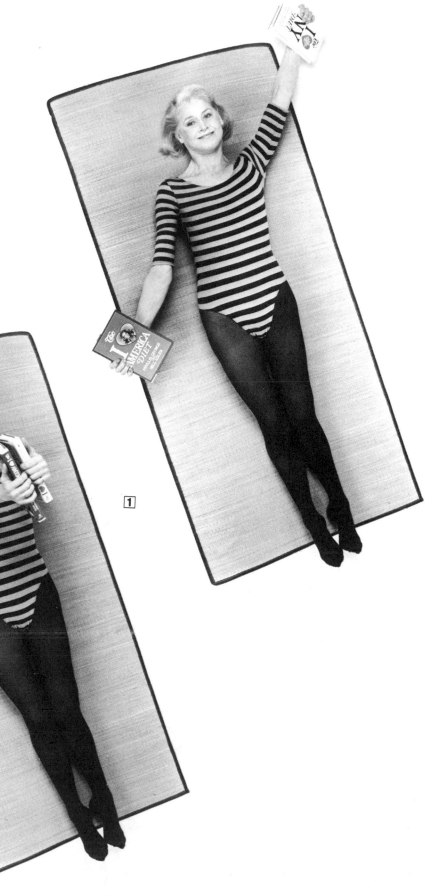

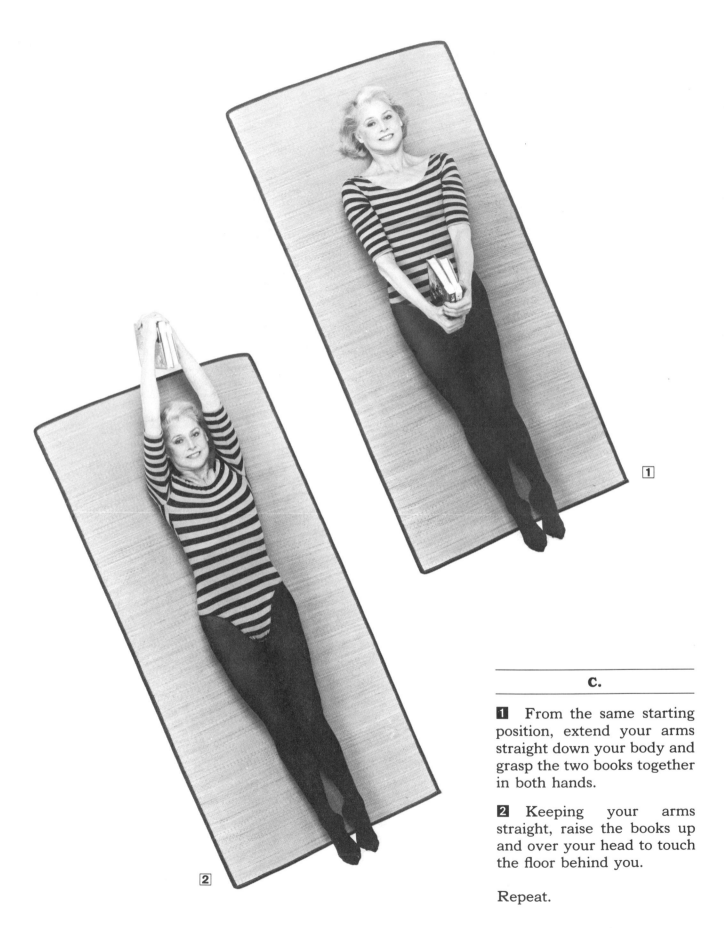

c.

1 From the same starting position, extend your arms straight down your body and grasp the two books together in both hands.

2 Keeping your arms straight, raise the books up and over your head to touch the floor behind you.

Repeat.

216

Heavy-Duty Rovers

My Super-Mom does this exercise with weights on her ankle, but you might want to build up to that gradually.

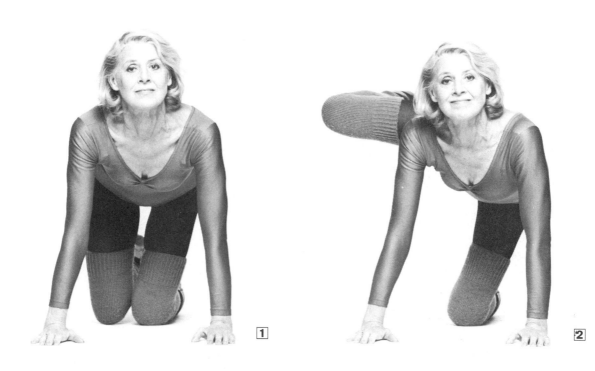

1 Start on all fours, with knees and feet together, arms straight and palms flat on floor, fingers pointing forward.

2 Lift your right leg up and out to the side at right angles to your body, keeping your knee bent and toes pointed.

3 Straighten your leg out and up to the side, as high as you can. And again.

4 Repeat the exercise with your left leg.

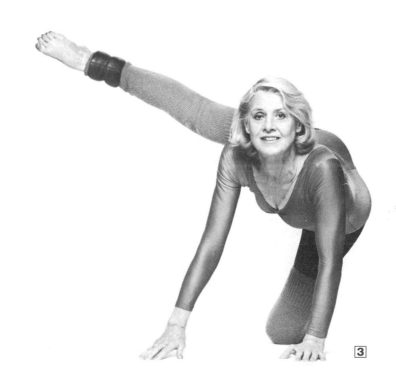

Side Splits

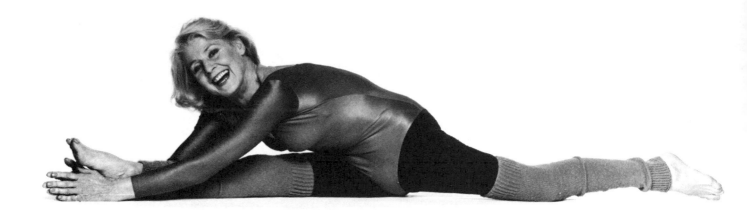

1 In split position, reach out for your right foot, with your forearms on the floor on either side of your leg, bringing your head down until it touches your leg.

2 Repeat, reaching out to your left foot; then alternate.

Mom-and-Me Sit-Ups

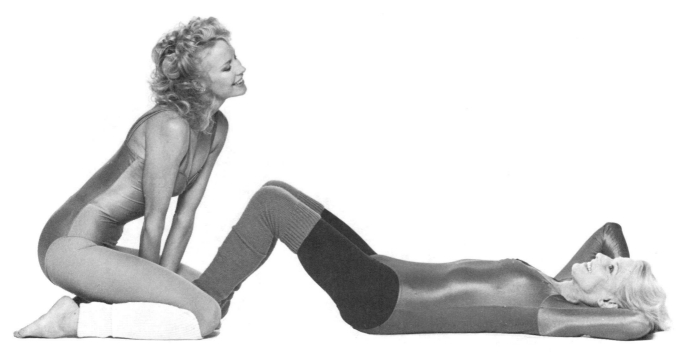

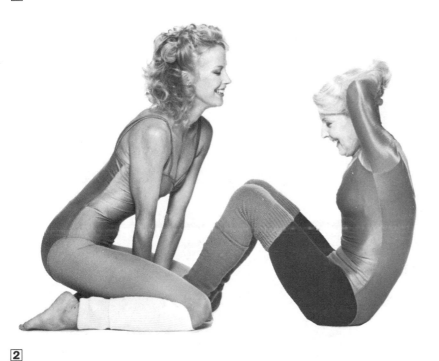

2

1 Lie on your back, arms folded beneath your head, knees bent up in an inverted V, with your daughter (or son, friend, or husband), holding your feet flat on the floor.

2 Using your daughter's hold as leverage, raise your body to a sitting position.

Repeat.

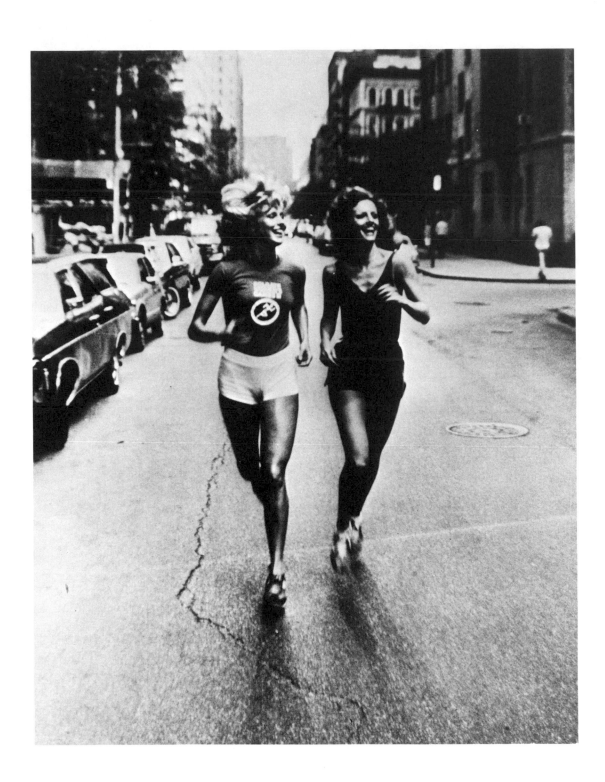

Don't Forget . . .

Exercising is wonderful, but it doesn't match the benefits of engaging in a sport you really love. Sports help you build energy, confidence, even friendships. They help you fight off the harmful effects of stress. They help you feel better, think better, become a better person. Women who engage in sports are more likely to reach their full potential than women who don't.

That's why I've been fighting for women's rights in sports for more than a decade, why I have lobbied Congress and four Presidents to initiate new programs benefiting women's athletics, why I serve on the boards of the President's Council on Fitness and Sports, the Women's Sports Foundation, and the Girl Scouts of America.

Many dedicated people have worked shoulder-to-shoulder with me, including Olympians Donna de Verona and Jack Kelly; and numerous sports-conscious legislators, Gerald Ford, Ted Kennedy, Tip O'Neill, Ted Stephens, and Bill Bradley among them, have recognized that sports mean better health, and women have as much right to better health as men.

If you can join the fight to support sports for women in your community, do it. And if you're not now enjoying the sport of your choice, start today. *The I Love New York Fitness Program* has readied you for it.